The 28 Day Gut Kickstart: Reinvent the Way Your Body Looks, Moves, Feels & Thinks

By Dr. Lauryn Lax

Copyright © 2018 by Dr. Lauryn Lax.

All rights reserved. No part of this publication may be reproduced, distributed, or transmitted in any form or by any means, including photocopying, recording, or other electronic or mechanical methods, without the prior written permission of the publisher, except in the case of brief quotations embodied in critical reviews and certain other noncommercial uses permitted by copyright law. For permission requests, write to the author at the address below.

lauryn@drlauryn.com

Edited by Jyssica Schwartz

www.jyssicaschwartz.com

Dedication

To Cathy, who first opened my mind to begin my own Gut Kickstart. To Meg, my "sister in crime" in the mission of helping others take back their health through simple medicine. To mom and dad, who always believed in me and affirmed me of my worth, at my core. And to those on their own healing journeys, inside and out.

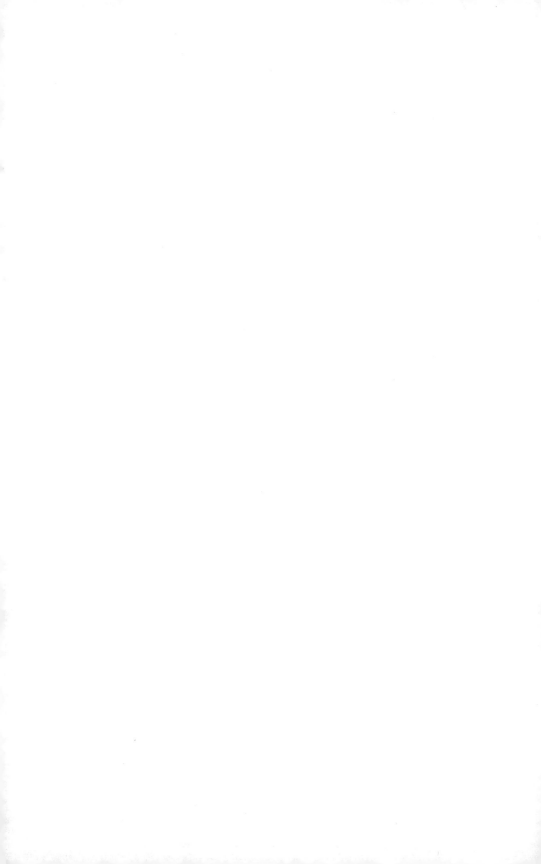

Table of Contents

Introduction: Love Your Gut 7

Chapter 1: Big Macs Are NOT Normal 17

Chapter 2: What 26 Years of Processed Food Does
          to Your Body 29

Chapter 3: Picture Perfect: What Ideal Digestion &
          Health Looks Like 35

Chapter 4: Digestion Gone Wrong: Leaky Gut 101 49

Chapter 5: Beyond Leaky Gut: 8 Reasons Why Your
          Gut is Imbalanced 57
    Low Stomach Acid 58
    Food Intolerances 60
    SIBO (Small Intestinal Bacterial Overgrowth) 68
    Infections (Parasitic & Bacterial) 71
    Disrupted Gut Bacteria (Dysbiosis) 75
    Toxic Burden (Liver & Gallbladder Dysfunction) 78
    Structural Imbalances 81
    Lack of "Gut Love" 86

Chapter 6: Dancing with Pink Elephants:
          Addressing Stress 89
    The Stress-Gut Connection 94
    Stress & Gut Love Assessment 137

Gut Check-In Point 140

Chapter 7: Gut Kickstart **141**
    Phase 1: Assess, Don't Guess 145
    Phase 2: Establish a Base 205
    Phase 3: Add in Gut Healing 275

Chapter 8: The Secret Sauce (Gut Love)............................**285**

Chapter 9: Get Started: Your 28-Day Gut Kickstart...........**289**

Gut Love Resources **295**
    Complete Gut Kickstart Food List........................304
    Cheat Sheet Protocols: Constipation, Bloating,
    Allergies & Everything in Between! 356
    FAQS...403

Resources/References **411**

Author Bio **427**

INTRODUCTION

Love Your Gut

Do you remember your first-ever "most embarrassing" moment?

That time in your life when you first realized what shame around an awkward happening overwhelmed you?

I was 6 years old at Vacation Bible School, and during circle story time I let one rip.

Immediately growing red-faced, the other kids in the classroom burst out in laughter, while they all diverted away from me to the outer edges of the story time carpet—leaving me alone in the middle, like Pumba in *The Lion King*.

"Lauryn tooted!" one of the little boys snickered.

Mortified, the bible teacher attempted to hush us back down and redirect attention to *Noah's Ark*, however, from that time forward, I knew what embarrassment was—and I also knew I had something funky going on in my gut.

Life continued on, but so did my own gut "issues."

TUMS Are Candy
Growing up, I popped TUMS like candy.

Mom kept them on tap in the medicine cabinet and in her purse. Any time I complained of a tummy ache, the soothing acid-reduction powers of my assorted berry and tropical orange tablets came to the rescue.

My pediatrician Dr. Joe told me I had an enlarged intestine during a routine check-up when my mom brought me in because she was concerned I wasn't pooping—constantly constipated.

For the latter part of that year, I ate "special" Fiber One cereal with strawberries every morning for breakfast. The kind that tasted like sticks. Some weeks, mom bought Frosted Mini Wheats. Those were special weeks. She also packed boxes of raisins, Fiber One granola bars, and dried prunes and apricots for snacks.

But still, not much got better.

Fast forward to middle school, when I began struggling with food and eating disorders, being told what to eat became my norm. Mom and dad took me to doctors and nutritionists who told me my "medicine" was to eat more cheese and milk, whole grains and normal teen foods like pizza and ice cream, and focus less on eating "safe foods" like vegetables and fruits.

In eating disorder treatment, my diet and malnutrition was supplemented with Ben & Jerry's, Snickers bars, Teddy Grahams with chocolate milk, packaged peanut butter crackers, Papa John's pizza, Doritos chips, Poptarts, Twinkies, Boost and Ensure weight gain shakes, and an extra roll with margarine at dinner.

Throughout the rest of my middle school, high school and early college years, these recommendations and prescriptions continued as professionals tried to help me recover from the extremist diet-mentality. The method? Exposure therapy: Challenge upon challenge to eat processed, packaged and "normal" foods from the Standard American Diet to help "desensitize" my food rules. Nonetheless, my "gut feelings" were rarely accurate in their eyes. If I voiced, "I don't feel well" or "my stomach really hurts" after eating pizza and a milkshake or shrimp fettuccine Alfredo, many of my dietitians and recovery coaches told me, "It's all in your head," or "That's the eating disorder speaking."

They were somewhat right. Processed junk foods were not my eating disorder's cup of tea.

However, even in my stretches of my "I will recover" motivation and mindset, I *still* didn't feel well for many years under the guise of these protocols. Constipation, bloating, IBS, and gas were my norm —continually doctored and suppressed with more TUMS, Pepto Bismol, and Miralax. "Just take this," nurses and doctors told me, never questioning or addressing the root issues. WHY was I constipated, gassy or bloated, ALL the time?

In a fit of violent rage at the nutrition "therapy" administered to me in the hospital during one of my many stays, my body fought back—contracting a parasite that left me soiling myself or throwing up involuntarily for three days straight before the doctors figured out what was up through testing. The prescription? Antibiotics and "upping" my meal plan to replace the lost calories and electrolytes in the mess— not one, but two Poptarts with breakfast, an extra Boost shake with my chicken nuggets, Coca Cola and French fries at lunchtime, and some ice cream to top off my spaghetti and meat sauce with buttered garlic bread at dinner.

While many other times and instances are blurry, what I most remember from the first 24 years of my life is my body being at war with itself—living in one of two extreme worlds:

1. The Standard American Diet—Processed and packaged foods. Fast foods and takeout. An emphasis on calories, not food quality.
2. The Diet Mentality—Diet rules and diet foods galore: diet bars, diet shakes, raw vegetables, juices, no meat diets, low-fat diets, low calorie diets, no carb diets, all-protein diets, 'eating clean' (egg-whites only) bodybuilding diets. *Anything* to be "healthy" (at least according to the diet world's standards).

The universal theme of both? The constipation, bloating, abdominal cramping, and gas persisted.

Neither dietary philosophy made me feel well (Even when I was following "the rules" by either dietitians or the diet world's standards). Something was not right. In addition, I suffered from osteoporosis, malabsorption, low Vitamin D, anxiety, skin rashes and breakouts, annual sore throats and colds, and blood sugar imbalances (getting shaky or hungry between meals)—so much so that I resolved "I suppose this is my normal."

Guess what? **It is NOT.** None of the symptoms I experienced for the first 24 years of my life were normal—or at least they did not have to be.

The Straw That Broke the Camel's Back
My "aha" moment or lightbulb moment that I didn't have to feel this way came the day I drank a pitcher of Crystal Light. Make that two.

On the cusp of age 24, in graduate school, eating "on-the-go" was a regular routine. Since I didn't eat much at the time (about 5 different foods), I relied on Crystal Light to fill me up and keep me going. Every day I'd fill up my 32 ounce Nalgene bottle with the Tropical Strawberry-Banana-Orange delight and tote it to class to keep me from getting hungry and thinking about food instead of neuroanatomy. I'd savor it throughout the day—half a bottle with breakfast and half a bottle with lunch. The perfect sweet treat to top off my protein shake with 15 almonds and dry turkey patty and steamed zucchini meals.

One particular day however, I decided to pack two Nalgene bottles. Two Nalgene bottles with a total of 64 ounces of Crystal Light, instead of 32 ounces. Come 5pm, after class, I found myself on all fours on the floor of my apartment—praying to God that I'd never drink Crystal Light again if He'd just make the stabbing, shooting, chronic, throbbing pains go away. My intestines coiled and screamed to be free, and my tummy ballooned like a beach ball as I laid on the floor.

Why is this happening?

For whatever reason, I'd never put two and two together—connecting my former gas, bloating, headaches, blurred vision and nausea I sometimes felt during the days I drank my pitchers of Crystal Light. But this day, writhing in pain, the only thing I could chalk it up to was the double dose of artificial sweet goodness.

It was then and there I realized, perhaps **I didn't have to feel this way**. Perhaps my body didn't have to be at war with itself. And perhaps there was something to not only the food i was feeding my body, but also something to how I had been treating my body and connecting to my body for the previous 24 years of my life.

The same thing goes for YOU too.

YOUR GUT STORY

While this story is my story, it's *not* just my story.

Although there are no hard statistics around just how many people are actually struggling with "gut" issues (since many of them go undiagnosed), it is estimated that 3 in 4 Americans—75% of people—have some form of GI "dysfunction." Moreover, regular gas, bloating, GERD, constipation or other symptoms are not always correlated with gut health or function.

Other common signs and symptoms of "gut issues" include things like:

- Skin breakouts and acne
- Seasonal allergies

- Low immunity
- Fatigue
- Thyroid disorders
- Anxiety
- Depression
- OCD
- ADD/ADHD
- Difficulty concentrating or "brain fog"
- Cravings for caffeine or sugar
- Unwanted weight gain or weight loss
- "Stubborn metabolism"
- Autoimmune diseases
- Chronic headaches and Migraines
- Autism and sensory processing disorders
- Cancer
- Heart disease
- Frequent illness (always get colds or feel under the weather)
- Can't hold correction or adjustments (chiropractor)
- Diabetes
- Blood sugar imbalances
- Gout,
- Hormone imbalances (PMS, PCOS, infertility)
- Poor gym performance and recovery

The struggle is real. A vast majority of the chronic and acute diseases that plague us today can be attributed back to our gut health and the integrity of our gut lining.

Hard Work

Perhaps it sounds simplistic, but if you think about it: *What organ and body system is responsible for delivering every single nutrient and filtering every single toxin you ingest or come into contact with throughout your life?*

Your gut.

Moreover, which body system works just as hard as your heart or your brain to keep you alive and well?

Your gut (it's what is responsible for feeding you!).

On average, your gut intercepts at least three meals per day—and goes to work:

1. Breaking down food in your mouth
2. Acidifying it in your stomach
3. Passing it on to your small intestine
4. Distributing nutrients (or toxins) through your bloodstream
5. Processing and detoxifying any outside invaders (pollutants, pesticides, sugars, mold, etc.) which got lumped in there with your spinach salad
6. Creating bulk and waste from anything it doesn't want
7. Eventually spitting it out of your other end

It's a complex process which can take up to 48-72 hours per meal for some, so if something is awry in the system or process, that is where disease (and these signs and symptoms of GI dysfunction) may arise.

"Leaky gut" is a popular term we will get more into later, but essentially, when we eat foods our body does NOT recognize as real food (processed, packaged, refined foods) OR when we are exposed to repetitive stressors (i.e. antibiotics, smoke, toxic hygiene, mental stress, circadian rhythm dysfunction, and cleaning products, mold, etc.) our gut takes a hit.

Yes, the struggle is real.

What to Do About It

In the following pages, we are going to explore your own gut story and address these four primary points:

1. **What is Normal?** First, we'll begin with questioning what "norms" you have settled for in your health that are actually *not* normal? Your acne? Pollen allergy? Bloating or gas after most meals? Constipation several days in a row? Needing coffee for energy? ADD or ADHD?

2. **Picture Perfect Digestion.** From there we'll move on to a basic understanding of what ideal gut health and digestion is in the first place and clear up some common buzz phrases like "leaky gut," probiotics, and gut bacteria.

3. **Underlying Gut Issues.** Then we'll dive into the seven primary gut pathologies, or root causes, of most gut issues. Unlike conventional medicine and insurance which acknowledges and treats gut symptoms like IBS, constipation, acne and GERD, you're going to find out what causes these symptoms in the first place in order to address the symptoms and heal (not manage) your gut.

4. **Customized Gut Kickstart Protocols & Lifestyle Gamechangers.** Lastly, we will have a heart-to-heart about "what to do about it." Instead of giving you a TON of information, I'm going to give you the inside scoop to assessing, testing, healing, and treating—not just managing—your symptoms and root issues. This includes a 28 Day Gut Kickstart you can start to give you the practical play-by-play steps for "getting there."

No matter where you are in your gut healing journey, there is more for you. Your body was meant to feel good. Really good. (In fact, you probably don't know how amazing you *can* feel).

It's time to write a new gut story, end the war in your own skin, and reinvent the way you look, move, think and feel. It's time to love your gut.

CHAPTER 1

Big Macs Are NOT Normal

I'm Not Lovin' It…

"Do you want fries with that?"

No, I didn't want fries. But as part of my therapy and treatment, my nutritionist wanted me to get fries.

"Yes. Fries, please."

Scene: McDonald's. Fast food challenge restaurant outing in treatment. I'd earned the privilege to venture outside the four walls of eating disorder treatment with the body-image therapist. On this particular day, McDonald's was on the agenda. My nemesis.

Founded in 1948 by the McDonald brothers, McDonald's changed the game of eating in America. Although a couple of other fast food chains were established prior (White Castle and A & W), McDonald's is credited with scaling fast food to a multi-national level, with over 30,000 franchises worldwide today, and with taking grain-fed meat from "good" to "great" in the name of convenience, wallet savings, and *fast* food. And, while we can all acknowledge fast food is not that "great" for us—low in nutrients—we can also all acknowledge that Big Macs and French fries (along with sub sandwiches, packaged snack bars, snack crackers, chips and dip, diet soda, cereal, takeout pizza, sugar-free ice cream, and other additive-rich foods) have all become "norms" in our society.

But is McDonald's *really* normal?

Reality Check

Walk into any McDonald's and ask where they source their meat and chances are you'll hear, "It's shipped in every morning at 5 a.m." or "Ummm…McDonald's?" In other words, they don't really know.

McDonald's (and other fast food chains) gets their frozen burger patties from about 20 different food processing companies with beef from 400,000 different beef suppliers worldwide, raising CAFO (concentrated agricultural feeding operation) cows. **Read**: antibiotics, hormones and bacteria. Not only is this horrible for the animals and the environment, but eating meat from sick animals can make you sick.

Not to mention the multiple at-home experiments on "McDonald's hamburgers that don't rot."

It all started back in 2008, when Karen Hanrahan shared a photograph of a McDonald's hamburger she bought 12 years earlier (in 1996) on her blog, Best of Mother Earth. The 12-year-old burger looked nearly identical to a fresh McDonald's burger. Since then, YouTubers and bloggers alike have posted viral pictures of dry burger patties that "don't go bad." Why not? The burgers—like shelf-stable crackers, beef jerky, and hockey pucks—dry out. (Imagine what happens in your gut).

Couple this with the additive-rich buns, containing ingredients such as:

The 28 Day Gut Kickstart

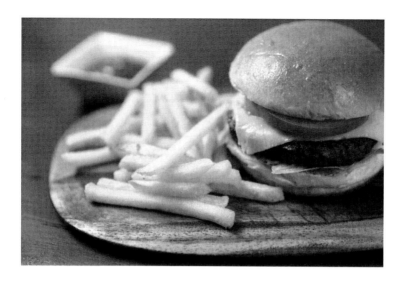

Enriched flour (bleached wheat flour, malted barley flour, niacin, reduced iron, thiamine mononitrate, riboflavin, folic acid), water, high fructose corn syrup and/or sugar, yeast, soybean oil and/or canola oil, contains 2% or less of the following: salt, wheat gluten, calcium sulfate, calcium carbonate, ammonium sulfate, ammonium chloride, dough conditioners (may contain one or more of the following: sodium stearoyl lactylate, datem, ascorbic acid, azodicarbonamide, mono- and diglycerides, ethoxylated monoglycerides, monocalcium phosphate, enzymes, guar gum, calcium peroxide), sorbic acid, calcium propionate and/or sodium propionate (preservatives), soy lecithin.

- **Ammonium Chloride.** Used in fireworks and explosives.
- **Ammonium Sulfate.** Used as an artificial fertilizer and in flame retardant materials.
- **Enriched flour.** i.e. nutrition taken out, and replaced with difficult-to-digest refined flours.
- **Soybean and canola oil.** Hydrogenated oils associated with inflammation, elevated cholesterol, and heart disease and cancer-causing agents

Along with ketchup, infused with:

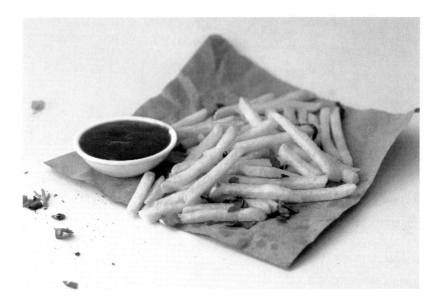

Ingredients: Tomato concentrate from red ripe tomatoes, distilled vinegar, high fructose corn syrup, corn syrup, water, salt, natural flavors (vegetable source)

Fact: Most corn or corn syrup is GMO—genetically modified organisms - associated with massive tumors in rats. During a two-year study (Seralini et al, 2014) originally published in the journal Food and Chemical Toxicology, researchers discovered that rats fed Monsanto's "Roundup Ready" corn and GMO foods developed aggressive tumors and died sooner than rats in the control group (70 percent GMO fed rats vs. 20-percent non-GMO fed rats). Furthermore, the tumors of rats of both sexes fed genetically-modified corn were two to three times bigger than rats not fed the same corn.

McDonald's Isn't the Only Culprit

McDonald's is not the only culprit when it comes to foods and lifestyle behaviors of modern day considered "normal," but are really not normal.

From staring at screens 7-10 hours per day, drinking diet soda and coffee as "water," consuming artificial sweeteners (including stevia), lack of light exposure during the day (and lots of blue light at night), and other processed foods (even "healthy" gluten-free products), our modern day lifestyles are far from the "norms" of our natural-born wiring.

In fact, did you know that 80 percent of foods sold in the grocery stores are man made, processed food-like products—representing the majority of Americans' diets? From Goldfish crackers to protein powders and bars, diet sodas, whole grain breads, fruit-on-the-bottom yogurt, chips, frozen dinners, gluten-free crackers, processed and packaged man made, food-like products have become "norms" in society, too.

But…are processed foods *really* normal for humans to eat? Technically, no.

While the average "normal" 21st century human eats many of these foods (and my therapist told me eating French fries and a Big Mac were "normal" during the fast food McDonald's challenge), our innate human biology was not wired or designed to *survive* or *thrive* off these foods.

Just like if you were to water a plant with gasoline or fill the tank of a Ferrari with water, they would not function ideally; the human body does not function ideally when we lack real foods.

Sure, adaptation *can* happen to our environment *and* we cannot live in bubbles (i.e. perfection is impossible), but "normal eating" (per society's standards) leads to major health side effects.

Gut issues work the same way. They are considered "normal," but they really are not normal - or they don't have to be.

Gut Issues Are Not Normal

We are currently in one of the worst epidemics of humankind time. One in two adults and one in two kids have one or more chronic disease—classified as any disease or health issue which has persisted for three or more months.

People in the 21st century face health conditions no other generation or human population experienced to such a large magnitude, including:

- Diabetes & blood sugar imbalances
- Weight management difficulties
- Rheumatoid arthritis
- Autism
- ADD/ADHD
- Depression
- Chronic fatigue syndrome
- Metabolic disturbances
- Hashimotos/Thyroid disorders
- Autoimmune diseases
- Anxiety
- Depression/Mood imbalances
- Eating disorders
- Acne
- Infertility, PCOS and PMS
- Heart disease
- Inflammation
- Gout
- High cholesterol
- Vitamin D deficiency

- Chronic ear infections, sore throats or other suppressed immunity
- Allergies
- Low immunity
- Cancer
- Alzheimer's and brain disease(s)
- Skin breakouts and acne

Despite our awareness, however, projection for rates of these diseases are only estimated to get worse—not better.

For instance:

- **Between 2000 and 2010, Autism rates experienced a 119 percent increase** in diagnosed cases, sending the prevalence rate to about 1 in every 68 kids (CDC, 2017).

- **Heart disease and cancer continue to be the leading causes of death in the country**—responsible for nearly 50% of all mortality combined (Weir et al, 2016).

- **One in three adults and one in six kids is overweight or obese** (NIDDK, 2017) **and the same stats apply to those with both diabetes and prediabetes** (CDC, 2017). Diabetes treatment alone costs the U.S. over $300 billion dollars every year (Diabetes Care Report, 2014). To put this in perspective, the estimated cost to cure world hunger is $30 billion dollars every year, according to the United Nations (Laborde et al, 2016).

- **Approximately one in five people suffer from a mental illness, such as eating disorders, anxiety and depression** (AMI, 2015), and SSRIs are the third most frequently taken medication in the U.S. with about 1 in 10 people on an antidepressant (Pratt et al, 2011).

- **One in three seniors dies with Alzheimer's or dementia** and prevalence of the disease will triple by 2050 (AA, 2017)
- **Nearly 50% of all adults have "adult acne"** (Collier et al, 2008)—a condition which is most often chalked up to genetics or your skin care routine, even though the skin care beauty industry is close to generating $100 billion each year in sales on everything from anti-aging creams to acne face wash and so many more (Lucintel, 2016).
- **Half of all people have allergies and sensitivities, including food intolerances, seasonal allergies or asthma.** (AAFA, 2017). Current medicine says they cannot explain this rise, but speculate the "hygiene hypothesis" to be the driving force— a **hypothesis** which states "lack of early childhood exposure to infectious agents, symbiotic microorganisms (such as the gut flora or probiotics), and parasites increases susceptibility to allergies by suppressing the development of the immune system." Translation: People do not have enough healthy gut bacteria based on a lack of exposure as a child.

Old News
Yawn.

More than likely, stats such as these fall on deaf ears. We've heard them all before. And yet, because they are so normal in our society, it's easy to chalk chronic disease up to being "normal."

Newsflash: They are not. Or at least they don't have to be.

"But it's in my genetics! It IS my norm," you say.

Even if your health condition(s) (or lack thereof) is similar to something your mom, dad, grandpa or grandma had, genetics only contribute to 5-10 percent of overall disease and health. The other 90-95 percent? Lifestyle and your gut health.

Believe it or not, all of these conditions stem back to your gut health.

Your Gut is the Gateway
Your gut health is the gateway to and the epicenter of your health—the core through which all of your nutrients and toxins must pass (throughout your entire life).

Over time, if the gut experiences "wear and tear" (***when** it experiences wear and tear),* from outside forces (poor quality foods, toxic burden, high stress lifestyles, etc.), then breakdown happens.

Why?

Your gut is what feeds and nourishes your entire body! However, if it's unable to feed and nourish your body to the best of its ability, diseases such as those listed above and imbalances are a given.

Given the approximation that at least one in two people have some sort of diagnosed chronic disease, not to mention the undiagnosed rate of individuals who experience symptoms like allergies, acne, headaches, rashes, thyroid and hormone imbalances (infertility, horrible PMS, PCOS, etc.) on the regular, we *must* look to the state of our gut health and whether your body is being fed and digesting your nutrients appropriately.

Moreover, if you have a gut imbalance, a vast majority of individuals may *not* experience the feeling of gut symptoms (bloating, constipation, GERD) at all—which is why many go **undiagnosed,** as many do not suspect a gut pathology to play a significant role in your health. ***In other words, "GI dysfunction" does not necessarily mean you feel bloated or constipated.***

What Causes GI "Dysfunction?!"
Good question.

One word: Stress. Not just mental stress. Physical stress as well. Common stressors we encounter throughout our lifetime include:

- Processed and packaged foods
- Processed diet foods
- Hydrogenated vegetable oils (found in many restaurant foods)
- Sugar—snuck in thousands of foods
- Conventional meats and dairy, administered antibiotics and hormones
- GMOs and pesticides in our vegetables and fruits
- Harsh chemicals and toxins in our cleaning and hygiene products
- Medications, including NSAIDs
- Antibiotics
- Polluted or toxin-filled water sources
- Frequent use of plastics and tupperware containers
- Travel out of the country to less developed ones—exposure
- Chemical and environmental pollutants
- Dietary influence—the amount, type, and balance of proteins, fats, carbohydrates, fiber, and fermentable carbohydrates that we eat or don't eat
- Physical inactivity **or** overtraining
- Mental stress (i.e. the brain-gut connection)
- Not listening to our body (i.e. not taking the time to go to the bathroom, neglecting our feelings of indigestion when we eat certain foods, etc.)
- Circadian rhythm disruption (i.e. blue light at night from screens, not sleeping enough, etc)
- Not chewing our food or slowing down when we eat

- A history of being a C-section or formula-fed baby can also contribute to a lifetime of gut issues

Exhibit A

When I discovered just how much lifestyle stressors play a role in gut health alone, ALL of my years of chronic "gut issues" finally made sense.

- I ate a steady diet of processed and packaged foods as a kid (I never saw a vegetable outside my broccoli and cheese sauce or canned green beans)
- Many doses of antibiotics for chronic ear and throat infections
- Thousands of harsh chemicals in cleaning and hygiene products from Walmart and Target
- Elevated screen time as I grew older
- Drinking from many plastic water bottles
- Rushing through my meals or mindlessly watching TV while I ate
- Lack of real foods and real fiber (vegetables) in my diet
- Chronic dieting and abuse of my body through over-training and a steady diet of fake protein bars and shakes for over 15 years

It wasn't until discovering the truths I am going to share with you in the following pages that I said, *"Hmmm…No wonder my gut (and my health) was not right."*

Long story short: Your body and health imbalances and "gut issues" may be considered "normal" by society's standards, BUT, just like Big Macs are technically NOT normal, these things do not have to be either.

CHAPTER 2

What 26 Years of Processed Food Does to Your Body

"Please help me go, please help me go" —a breathy prayer I often said out loud in the pit of discomfort, just wanting (and needing) to "go," but NOT being able to just "go" for days.

Stuck—often times how I felt in my own skin. Stuck in my gut. Constipated. Like my body was at war with itself.

At age 26, even though I ate "healthy" (on paper), something was not right.

Greens? Check.
Sweet potatoes? Check.
Salmon? Check.
Almonds? Check.
Eggs? Check.
Broccoli? Check.
Coconut butter and coconut oil? Check.

I was doing ALL the "right things," so why did it have to hurt so much?

Answer: Being healthy goes far beyond diet alone. At least once you've been enlightened…

Day 1 Nutrition School: You Are Not Alone
"Stand up and introduce yourself. What got you interested in studying nutrition?" the teacher said.

One by one, my class of about 40 other aspiring nutrition therapy practitioners had to stand up and give their "elevator speech" as to why we were all sitting upright in the classroom, pen and paper in hand, eager, anxious and beaming with BIG vision, to learn how to save the world one food myth at a time.

As we went around the room sharing our stories, one by one, we each began to realize that…we were not alone.

Many of my fellow classmates were survivors of the processed-food, antibiotic, vaccine, sedentary lifestyle and chronic disease generation, and somehow had all lived to tell about it.

"My son was diagnosed with Autism, and the doctors told me there was nothing we could do about it except lots of therapies and behavior plans. So I did some research myself, and began to find stories about the brain-gut connection—how food can influence how we think and help kids with Autism. As a family, we started the GAPS diet, and my son, who was non-verbal, said his first words," Charlotte said.

"I was a vegetarian and vegan for over 15 years, and on the cusp of my 30th birthday, I got sick—really sick," Lynan said. "My skin was pale, my hair started falling out, my nails were brittle, I was tired all the time, lost my period, and began experiencing bloating around meals all the time. Something wasn't right. I thought it was something to do with my hormones, or maybe mono or anemia, so I went to a doctor a friend recommended and he said nothing was wrong with me. I just needed to eat meat again, telling me, "You know you are doing the same thing to your body that inhumane chicken and beef farms do to their animals—feeding them lots of grains and processed foods, restricting them from all the nutrients their bodies need to thrive. Your body needs balance." I was so desperate for anything to feel better, so I gave it a try, and within a matter of months, all my health problems went away. I got my period and energy back, the bloating subsided and I felt better than I had in those 15 years," Lynan said.

"I got terminal brain cancer. The doctors gave me 2, maybe 3 months to live, and told me it had spread through every bone in my body and that there was nothing I could do," Bob said, "But then I looked on the nutrition label of the tube-feeding formula the healthcare company sent me, only to see the words 'Nestle' and 'high fructose corn syrup' on the 'medicine' meant to help me get the extra nutrients I needed, and I thought, 'There's got to be another way.' So I decided to start juicing my own food and smoothies for my feeding tube, and just ate real food. Months later, I was completely cancer free and years later, I have a son they told me I could never have and I lived to tell about it. I want to help people," Bob said.

Mic drop.

Nope. None of us were alone.

What 26 Years of Processed Foods Does to Your Body
We all have a story. Often, multiple stories which shape us for the better or worse. Your stories are written via your life experiences, and chances are, when it comes to your health, you've had multiple experiences which have set the stage for where your body (and health markers) are today.

Even if you "eat healthy" and "do all the right things" today, your *past* experiences paved way for the way you feel (or don't feel) now.

I'm a Survivor

Hi, I am Lauryn and I am a survivor of the processed foods, take-a-Tylenol (Tums or antibiotic) for everything, drink-juice-as-water, frozen broccoli (with cheese sauce), Lean Cuisine and Quest Bars convenience (and health conscious) generation.

For the first 26 years of my life, my body didn't see a real food—really.

Sure, I ate Fiber One cereal and not Cookie Crisp for breakfast. I packed 99% lean turkey on whole wheat bread with pretzels (not chips) for lunch (with the special occasion Pizza Lunchable). Noshed on apple slices with peanut butter, or string cheese and whole grain Wheat Thins between meals, and I ate a low-fat dinner, including protein, starch, and veggies with a glass of milk most nights for dinner…but even though I was eating "healthy," (according to Standard American Diet criteria), my body did not see **real** food.

Fast forward to my teenage and college years when I began to make my own food choices for myself. I looked to magazines, social media, and Google for advice on what to eat (and not eat), following hundreds of food rules. If it was deemed "healthy" or "clean" by *Shape* or *Cosmo*, it was okay with me, including protein bars and powders, frozen dinners, raw veggies, tons of nuts and almond butter, egg white omelets, and no carbs, no meats or no fats (depending on the popular trend at the time).

Eating disorder treatment was a whole other can of worms complicating the story. Over the accumulated three years of my life spent in **inpatient** treatment centers and hospitals, along with 15 years of meal plans with prescriptions to eat McDonald's Egg McMuffins and Dairy Queen Blizzards, I just did not see (or eat) a real food—at least not much of it.

The universal theme? My body—namely my gut—didn't know how to deal with the influx of foods that were difficult to digest. The result? **A host of inflammation and imbalances.**

Even though I found "real food" at 26, and I was well beyond my eating disorder and had discovered the art of "stressing less," I had A LOT of damage to heal and make up for from the previous 26 years of my life.

In short: How you feel today (or how you will feel tomorrow or 50 years from now) is a result of the choices you made years ago and now.

Survey Says

I spent my entire 26th year of life studying nutrition and forming the foundations of my current functional medicine, nutrition and therapy business. The next year, I found myself in two rigorous functional medicine trainings and sinking my teeth (and brain) into anything that could explain more about WHY I felt the way I felt (i.e. constipated and bloated ALL the time), trying to understand WHY it seemed like no doctor could/would help me just feel good in my own skin. Instead of believing "bloating and constipation are just a part of life," I dedicated my studies and used my body as an experiment to find out if healing was truly possible.

The following results are from a few of my lab tests are just a glimpse of what 26 years of processed foods, lifestyle and gut stress does to your body.

Diagnosis: Osteoporosis:
Causes: Malnutrition, lack of essential fatty acids, inability to absorb nutrients ("leaky gut") and bacterial overgrowth.

Diagnosis: SIBO (Small Intestinal Bacterial Overgrowth):
Causes: High grain consumption, low stomach acid, stress, overtraining, artificial sweeteners, low-fat diets, FODMAP foods, antibiotics, processed and packaged foods.

Diagnosis: Colitis & Megacolon (inflammation of the Colon)
Causes: SIBO, parasites, low stomach acid, IBS, poor quality diet, serotonin

Diagnosis: High Cortisol (i.e. stress hormone):
Causes: "Leaky gut," overtraining (or sedentary lifestyle), lack of quality sleep, lack of water, burning the candle at both ends (trying to do it all), gut-inflammatory foods and food intolerances, high caffeine or sugar/artificial sweetener consumption, NOT going with your gut (and being true to yourself), LED light/screen exposure.

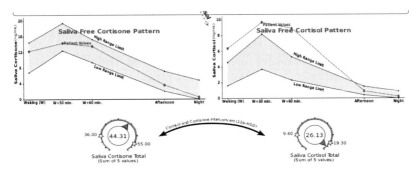

The Bottom Line

Knowledge is power and healing IS possible—even for me, with 26+ years of processed foods and other health stressors under my belt.

Before we start talking about what could be "wrong" with your own gut, let's get a clear picture of what **normal digestion** and **a healthy gut** (including your poop and passing gas) *should* look like.

CHAPTER 3

Picture Perfect: What Ideal Digestion & Health Looks Like

Your gut is the largest organ in your body.

The gastrointestinal or "GI" tract is a 30-foot hollow tube which technically starts in your mouth and ends in the anus. That's about the length of five refrigerators inside you!

It consists of the mouth, pharynx, esophagus, stomach, small intestine, large intestine, rectum, anus, and accessory organs that assist digestion, including the salivary glands, liver, gallbladder and pancreas.

The Jobs of Your Gut
The primary job of the GI tract is to break down the foods you eat, absorb the nutrients, and distribute them throughout your body—to your cells, muscles, bones, brain, organs and metabolic processes.

Second, the GI tract also serves as a "gatekeeper"—protecting you against antigens (i.e. foreign invaders) that want to leak into your bloodstream, outside the GI system, to take your body down.

While your gut may allow **nutrients OUTSIDE of the digestive tract** (to other parts of the body), it also puts up a fight to keep toxic wastes and foreign ingredients (chemicals, artificial sweeteners, pesticides, etc.) **OUTSIDE** of your bloodstream.

In short: everything that's kept **inside** your gut is actually **outside** of the body.

Sort of like a vault or safe in a bank that is PART of the bank, but they are kept "locked away" so they don't affect your overall health.

However, once foods, nutrients, toxins, or other foreign invader's get outside your gut (into your bloodstream), they affect your body's overall health, disease and nutrient status (for better or worse).

The Strength of Your Gut

Your gut lining is composed of four layers, which are a blend of connective tissues, muscle and fatty tissues: the mucosa, lamina propria, muscularis externa; and the outermost layer, the serosa/mesentery.

Translation: **Your gut is thick and strong**.

It takes A LOT of wear and tear for your gut to get worn out and let its guard down.

Nevertheless, if and when your gut faces *consistent* gut-irritating stressors (such as conventional meats, moldy toxin-filled coffee, antibiotics, long-term use of prescription medications or NSAIDS, artificial sweeteners, gut-irritating grains, soy, peanuts, toxic chemical beauty and cleaning products, under-eating, etc.) then your once strong gut lining becomes weaker.

Like lifting weights and working the same muscles *every* day makes you weaker and doesn't allow the muscles to rest and recuperate, when we overwork our gut lining with stressors we eat or put into/on our body without enough healthy gut-loving foods, we break it down over time.

In addition, things like bacterial overgrowth, fungal and parasitic infections and food intolerances may also arise. Hello constipation, bloating, nutrient deficiencies, mental anxiety, fatigue, thyroid imbalances, allergies, skin issues, hormonal imbalances, "genetic" health conditions, autoimmune disease, and other side effects galore!

So what does a "healthy gut" and "healthy digestion" actually look like?!

I'm so glad you asked!

Picture Perfect Gut Health
Your gut was designed to be one of the most sterile environments in the world.

Your "gut" refers to two primary components, your digestive tract and the organisms that live within the digestive system.

Part 1: Your digestive tract runs from your mouth to your colon, or anus, including the:

- Esophagus
- Stomach
- Small intestine
- Liver-gallbladder
- Pancreas (regulates blood sugar)
- Anus

Part 2: Your "gut microbiome," "microbiota" or "gut flora" —the organisms or 100 trillion bacteria that live INSIDE your digestive system. Fun fact: you have 10 times more bacteria than cells in your body—both good (commensal) and bad (pathogenic).

Your gut or "micro-biome" covers a surface area of about 400 m² (about 1/4th of a mile both deep and wide) and your gut barrier, or intestinal tissue lining, is strong and serves as a "gatekeeper" to keep toxins out of your blood stream, while allowing nutrients in and out to nourish all the cells in your body. To stay in tip-top shape, your gut requires about 40 percent of your body's energy expenditure—double the energy expenditure of your brain!

Layman's Terms
Think of your digestive system like the refrigerator and freezer in your home—with different jobs and shelves (ie. the freezer keeps things frozen, the crisper keeps veggies crisp, the top shelf is for leftovers, the side doors are for condiments, etc.).

Think of your gut microbiome, gut flora or gut bacteria as the different food items in your fridge and freezer—some good, and some not-so-good (depending on what you choose to fill your shelves with).

Sure, you keep healthy fruits and veggies in your fridge, but if you have more ice cream, Chinese takeout, and seven-day-old leftovers inside than you do real foods, your health will suffer over time. However, if you have many colorful fruits and veggies, organic meats and some healthy prepped meals on hand (consumed within about 3-4 days of prep), and a LITTLE bit of ice cream in the freezer, or one night's worth of takeout - then that's okay. Balance is good and moderation is important.

Even though the word "bacteria" may get a bad rep, your gut bacteria is actually REALLY GOOD for you. Picture perfect gut health includes a WIDE DIVERSITY of different strains of bacteria cultures to do some pretty amazing things, including:

- Support your immune system
- Digest your food

- Support mental clarity
- Assist with nutrient absorption
- Regulate your hormones
- Boost immune health and metabolism
- Normalizing glucose levels
- Support a healthy gut barrier
- Regulate inflammation
- Ward off pathogens and disease-causing microbes

In short: Gut bacteria do a body good…at least if they aren't stressed out or threatened by unhealthy lifestyle habits.

For Ideal Health, Look to Our Ancestors

Imagine if you had **NEVER** been raised to touch a processed food, sleep less than six hours each night, sit on a couch after work watching a screen or sit for eight hours at a desk hunched over, put chemicals used for furniture upholstery on your face, drink water with carcinogenic chemicals and only eat one or two veggies each day…

What do you think your health (and your gut health) would be like?

Sounds like the Garden of Eden, right? It's not.

Life without processed, packaged foods; screen exposure and isolation behind social media; pesticide-sprayed produce and conventionally raised meats; poor quality water **IS** the way humans lived since the beginning of time, prior to the Agricultural and Industrial Revolutions.

The human body was designed to live and thrive upon food from the Earth, connection to nature and others, and with ebbs and flows of stress.

In fact, a study (Smits et al, 2017) on the gut health of hunter-gatherer populations found that humans who live MOST IN TOUCH with our ancestors' way of life (eating real food, sleeping and rising with the sun, living in community with one another, not stressed over work deadlines, etc.) have MORE bacterial diversity in their guts and LESS disease. Despite their lack of access to medical care, they tend to live longer, healthier, and more productive lives.

Having a diverse microbiome helps us effectively defend ourselves from infections—unlike modern day Joe and Susan, who drink Starbucks coffee, work their sedentary 9-5 corporate America jobs, pop Advil to suppress headaches, and eat candy from the candy jar or fast-food salads in their car on the go to their son's soccer game.

Unfortunately, modern day life has presented a variety of forces working against your "ideal" health and digestion, which (in an ideal world) would look something like the following.

Step-By-Step: How Ideal Digestion is SUPPOSED to Work

STEP 1: Think & Taste Food.
The **normal** flow of digestion is a **north-to-south process.** Digestion starts in the brain, then goes to the mouth, in response to the thought, taste and appearance of food. Your salivary glands help produce enzymes to both digest carbohydrates and fight off microorganisms you may be exposed to. Chewing your food is crucial for activating these enzymes optimally.

STEP 2: Stomach.
From the mouth, food passes through the esophagus to the stomach—a J-shaped bag, where three main things happen:

- Short-term storage of food
- Mechanical and chemical breakdown of food **into chyme**—a paste-like substance (food mixed with stomach acid and enzymes)
- The killing of bacteria and foreign invaders that we swallow by the stomach acid

This process of making chyme and killing bacteria with stomach acid takes up to two hours, then the chyme moves to the small intestine, where the *majority* of digestion happens.

STEP 3A: Small Intestine.

The small intestine alone is about 18 feet (6 meters) in length and consists of three parts in descending order: the duodenum, the jejunum, and the ileum.

For the next 6-8 hours, your food (the chyme) is processed throughout this tract, where nutrients are absorbed and sent out to the appropriate cells, organs, muscles and metabolic processes needing them.

(Note: if you have a leaky gut OR bacterial overgrowth, the small intestine is often where GI dysfunction happens).

While digestion is happening in the small intestine, your body's accessory organs, including the **liver**, **gallbladder** and **pancreas** also go to work.

STEP 3B: Liver-Gallbladder-Pancreas

The **liver** is housed in the upper right region of your abdomen. Its main role in digestion is the filtering out of toxins, the production of bile (to help digest fats in your small intestine), and the distribution of nutrients.

ALL nutrients absorbed by the gut must pass through the liver to be processed before traveling through the rest of the body.

The **gallbladder** is the organ right below the liver which assists the liver in the storage and production of bile. If digestion is working properly, the gallbladder sends out bile every time you eat to the small intestine to help assist in the break down of your food.

Lastly, the **pancreas** is responsible for producing the enzymes which break down food in the small intestine—proteins, fats, and carbs included.

STEP 4: Large Intestine.
After your gut has done all the work it can do, it enters the large intestine for the final breakdown of any undigested food particles and fiber, as well as the production of waste (poo).

The large intestine consists of six sections approximately 4.5 feet in length including the appendix, the cecum, the ascending, transverse, descending and sigmoid colon, and the rectum.

It has three primary functions:

1. The creation of poo from any undigested foods
2. Digestion of some food by bacteria (bacteria feeding off of leftover wastes)
3. Reabsorption (recycling) of water, salts, carbohydrates, and vitamins for your body to use

After your large intestine has collected the remaining nutrients it can from any previously undigested foods, it sends everything out the back door, and is on alert for the next meal. Your gut is working 24/7.

STEP 5: The End.
From start to finish, *ideal* digestion take about 24-hours and any unwanted food particles or wastes end up in your poop (a "gold standard" indicator of how well you are digesting your food)..

What Does Your Poop Say About You?

- **Ideal: The Golden Nugget: Medium brown.** Solidly formed in the shape of an S or C. Passing 1-3 times per day.

  The following poo patterns are not ideal, and while ok on occasion, if these are regularly occurring, something is off with your poo, gut health and/or food.

- **Leftovers.** Can you see those Brussels sprouts, sweet potato or mushrooms you ate—and still not completely broken down? This is not ideal. Shows it did not pass through the entire process of digestion. Consider your food chewing practices.

- **Slip & Slide.** Watery and loose. Often times, you can see the foods you ate in this one too—semi-broken down. Watery stools usually mean you ate something that your body yells, "May day, May day! I don't like this." A hire incidence of increased "bad" bacteria is indicated and/or food intolerances.

- **Green Quease.** Green poo often with queasy feelings. May indicate your gallbladder is not thoroughly breaking down bile salts to move your poop to that brown color. Green poop is often provoked when we eat fattier foods, since bile helps break down fats too—like vegetable oils (canola, Crisco, processed olive oil) from restaurants, processed; greasy foods (Chinese takeout, a fast food burger or greasy slice of pizza); and even "healthy" fats (like coconut oil, butter, etc.).

- **Molding Clay.** If your stools are pale or clay-colored, you may have a problem with the drainage of your biliary system, which is comprised of your gallbladder, liver, and pancreas (similar to the Green Quease). Bile salts are released into your stools by your liver, giving the stoolsa brown color.

- **Mr. Stanky.** Dark, foul, sometimes greasy and/or stinky. Something's toxic (i.e. not right). Common toxin triggers include: Processed and refined foods. High amounts of non-organic, non-fresh foods and triggers. General toxicity overload. Additives and chemicals. Poor lifestyle habits (smoking, sedentary, fast food). Use of plastics.

- **The Big Dump.** After a day or two (or 3) of not going, you finally go...all at once. You wonder: How was that in there?! You struggle with constipation and moving bowels through, until it finally decides to come and dump, leaving you feeling cleansed. May indicate low stomach acid, sluggish motility and/or bacterial overgrowth.

- **Like a Rock.** Difficult to pass or rock like. You still get it out—but a little straining was included. Drink more water. And make sure you're eating your veggies—and the kinds your body likes (you may be eating lots of raw veggies for instance—which are harder to break down, or sensitive to FODMAPS—like broccoli and Brussels. Leafy greens—cooked down and sauteed—can be good for hard stools). In addition, assess the quality of your proteins and other foods (have you been eating processed meats or packaged food items—even "paleo" bars and crackers and breads?), as well as your fat intake—are you eating fats with your meals to help lubricate your digestive tract? Sometimes your body just needs some good ol' meat, veggies and healthy fats—and plenty of water—along with time to breathe, chew and enjoy your meals (not on the go).

❖ **Pellets**
Like acorns or little rocks, these come out in bits and pieces—in one setting, or throughout the day. Hard to pass and generally darker in color. Stress, low water intake, eating on the go, low fiber intake, low stomach acid and bacteria imbalance (low "good bacteria") all play leading roles in pellet poop. If you've experienced this, you're often thankful for whatever the poop gods will give you—but look to lifestyle factors to dig deeper and bring things up to speed with: apple cider vinegar in water before meals, pre-biotic and pro-biotic foods, some starchy veggies and plenty of greens, chewing your food and slowing down to breathe at meals, yoga and meditation—just to name a few.

Poo FAQ

What is poop anyway?
Poop, or feces, is a mixture of 75 percent water and the rest is dead bacteria that helped us digest our food along the digestive pathway, and other living bacteria, undigested food particles, fiber, and other wastes from food, cellular linings, fats, salts and substances released from the intestines and liver.

How often should I poop?
If you are eating three times per day and have a squeaky clean digestive system, you would be pooping anywhere from one to

two times per day of 'normal' formed stools—and feeling completely eliminated (i.e. not hard to pass, loose or watery, or bits and pieces). Think about how often your dog poops when you feed him or her? Typically shortly after the meal of the day, the dog needs to do the doo-doo. Same thing goes for you in an ideal world (no laxatives needed).

What does "healthy" poop look like?
An ideal, healthy poop should look sausage-like and be light brown in color. Sometimes it can be green if you ate green veggies—and that's okay, too! Veggies do a body good. However, if the stool is loose, watery *and* green, this is not always a healthy indicator—ie. diarrhea. It's ok if it's a little smelly—just not foul.

What is the average bowel transit time?
The average transit time for the meal you just ate (from start to finish) is about 12-24 hours if it's healthy. However, for some it can be anywhere from 24-72 hours (three days)…or shorter if "it's going straight through you."

What does it mean if I have loose, watery stools?
You're not digesting something appropriately—especially if there is a fast transit time. Loose, watery stools could indicate a bacterial overgrowth (like SIBO) in your upper bowel (small intestine), a lingering parasite in your digestive tract, or low HCL (stomach acid) to assist in the breakdown of food in the initial stages of digestion. Frequent bouts of diarrhea and loose stools may warrant diagnosis with IBD or IBS-D. Digging into the underlying issues could be the missing link in indicating why your stools continue to be watery, water stools happen occasionally, it may simply indicate that you ate your food too fast/didn't thoroughly chew it, you're stressed, or a particular food triggered the gut reaction (dairy, nuts, gluten, etc.).

What does it mean if I am constipated?
Something is awry. Bacterial overgrowth is a dominant stressor to the GI tract and may even result in IBS-Constipation (IBS-C). When bacteria from the large intestine build up in the small intestine in particular, it stalls the normal process of complete digestion. By the time wastes reach the large intestine, the timing has been delayed. Constipation also indicates you may not be drinking enough water, chewing your food appropriately, you're not eating enough fiber (or you're eating too much fiber), or you have food intolerances.

Does protein constipate me?
Too much of any one nutrient may constipate you. This is the reason we need a balance of all three—and a fallacy of many diets that eliminate one nutrient in particular (be it low-fat, low carb or low protein). Carbs—particularly veggies—add fiber to partner with fats and proteins and assist them down the digestive tract and add 'bulk' to stools. Fats lubricate your digestive system to make digestion possible. And proteins help promote more stomach acid in the stomach (necessary for all food breakdown) and are actually what help break down all foods in the body in the first place (in the form of enzymes like pepsin). Balance is key.

Why am I constipated when I travel?
Traveler's constipation happens when our body gets out of routine! We aren't eating our typical foods, going to the bathroom at our typical times, moving like we usually do, or taking our digestive aids—like probiotics—regularly. The result? Back up. It can take a few days—even a week—for traveler's constipation to resolve. In addition, airplane travel is extra dehydrating as we go up in the air in the plane—putting an extra stressor on the digestive system. Cure it: Pack your probiotics and digestive enzymes if you can, make sure to

drink plenty of water, walk—even if your routine is not happening -- and incorporate as many veggies as you can into your daily mix.

The Bottom Line

If you're experiencing health imbalances, OR your poop does not meet the "Gold Standard" on the poo chart, then we need to dig a little deeper (no pun intended), starting with "leaky gut."

CHAPTER 4

Digestion Gone Wrong: Leaky Gut 101

"Leaky gut" is a popular buzzword in health circles and gut speak, tossed around by nutritionists, Women's Health Magazine and Dr. Oz alike.

Pop question: What is it?

Let's start with the basics.

Your Gut Lining is Strong

The intestinal barrier (i.e. intestinal wall or gut lining) covers a surface of about 400 square meters and requires approximately 40 percent of the body's energy expenditure to keep food and other substances both in and out. It prevents against loss of water and electrolytes, as well as prevents the entry of antigens and microorganisms into the body. Your gut lining is also responsible for allowing the exchange of molecules between host and environment (like the lotion, makeup or essential oils you put on your skin) and absorption of nutrients in the diet.

Your gut lining has its job cut out for it (it's strong), except when it gets overworked or irritated.

Hello "leaky gut!"

Leaky Gut 101

Leaky gut, or "intestinal permeability" is a common "malfunction"—a leak that happens when you hit a speed bump or get a "nail in your tire," threatening ideal digestion. Some things which can cause this are:

- Not chewing your food thoroughly, eating too fast or in a hurry (preventing proper food breakdown)
- Frequently eating gut-irritating ingredients and chemicals your body DOESN'T recognize as "food" or can't easily digest (i.e. conventional meat with hormones and antibiotics, protein bars, high fructose corn syrup, artificial sweeteners, refined grains, soy, sugar, MSG, frozen dinners, hydrogenated oils like canola oil and grapeseed oil, etc.)
- Prescription medications, NSAIDS, and antibiotics
- Chronic stress (i.e. under-sleeping, overtraining, constant worry or anxiety, circadian rhythm dysfunction from things like screen light exposure nights or shift work, high caffeine and coffee consumption)
- Erratic or disordered eating habits (binging, purging, restriction, chronic under-eating, etc.)
- History of Infections or Illness (bacterial, virus, heavy metals, fungal overgrowth)
- Lack of fermented foods and fibers (probiotics and prebiotics, found in starchy tubers, root veggies and supplements like partially hydrolyzed guar gum)
- Toxic exposure (i.e. chemicals in beauty and cleaning products, plastics, carcinogens in water)
- Nutrient deficiencies (Vitamin A, Vitamin D, Short Chain Fatty Acids & Butyrate)
- Viral infections, surgeries and/or traumas to the body

- Other digestive issues we will discuss, like SIBO (small intestinal bacterial overgrowth), liver/gallbladder dysfunction, parasites, food intolerances, etc.

Over time, these stressors wreak havoc on your strong gut lining.

Imagine picking at a scab with your fingernail, over and over and over…What would happen?

Eventually it would get irritated and open. The same thing happens inside for your gut lining: eventually the gut lining loses its tight intestinal lining junctions that were once able to decide what **did** and **did not** escape outside your digestive tract.

The Result?
"Leaky gut."

Without tight junctions and its role as the "gatekeeper" of unnecessary particles out of the bloodstream, all hell breaks loose.

If "leaky gut" is present, food particles, toxins in our food, water and products, and other "foreign invaders" easily leak into the bloodstream, where your body responds with an "autoimmune attack" inside, attacking itself.

Enter: inflammation and a host of other side effects (Bischoff et al, 2014) like:

- Skin breakouts
- Food and seasonal allergies
- Brain fog, difficulty concentrating
- Hormone imbalances
- A "slow metabolism," unwanted weight gain/loss and blood sugar imbalances
- IBD & IBS
- Inflammatory diseases—like Diabetes, neurological and cognitive disorders, Alzheimer's, autoimmune disease,

Parkinson's, cancer, Arthritis, ADHD, autism spectrum disorders, fibromyalgia, and more (Bischoff et al, 2014).

The thing is: **You DON'T always feel "leaky gut" in your gut if you have it.**

Silent Leaky Gut Syndrome

You can be on a beach in Costa Rica, sipping Pina Coladas and listening to Jimmy Buffett songs, but if you rely on coffee every day, eat sugar occasionally, use Noxzema face cream wash, waiver between five and seven hours of sleep every night, and have a childhood history of antibiotics and processed food consumption, you're *still at risk* for unhealthy gut.

Get this: Upwards of 50 percent of relatives to family members with celiac disease (i.e. people who have a "leaky gut") do NOT have the same "gut symptoms" their family members with celiac disease do, but they ALSO test positive for "leaky gut" or "intestinal permeability" (Fasano et al, 2003/Rodrigo et al, 2017).

In other words, they have gut issues without feeling like they have gut "issues."

Although "leaky gut" used to be considered a "quack" philosophy in medicine or health research, today, more and more studies are pointing to **increased prevalence intestinal permeability** (leaky gut) as a **root cause** for many of our modern day epidemics—like obesity and Diabetes (Ohlsson et al, 2017), gestational diabetes during pregnancy (Mokkala et al, 2017), and essentially, *any* other "chronic inflammatory disease" (Sturgeon et al, 2017).

How do I know if I have it?

Good question! There are several signs that point to a leaky gut.

Sign 1: How Do You Feel?

The biggest marker of them all: How do you *feel?*

Leaky gut is highly linked to **other** signs of inflammation and diseases in your body.

From bloating and constipation, to non-gut based symptoms like chronic seasonal or environmental allergies to adult acne, achy and popping joints, chronic yeast infections, horrible migraines, crazy PMS, no period, thyroid dysfunction or a sluggish metabolism, there is a potential that leaky gut is present.

In addition to leaky gut or "intestinal permeability," there is also a bigger underlying GI issue or ongoing stressor at play (poor diet, chronic stress, poor sleep, etc.).

Common underlying issues we will further consider include: SIBO, parasitic infections, fungal overgrowth, low stomach acid and food intolerances. In fact, these underlying issues are often actually the real reason why leaky gut happens or persists in the first place.

As for stress—check in with your lifestyle. How is your nutrition? Your stress? Your sleep? If no bueno, then leaky gut has more room for potential.

YOU are your own best advocate for checking in with yourself and assessing…*how do you feel?*

Sign 2: Leaky Gut Testing

Lab testing can also help confirm the presence of "intestinal permeability."

To date, there are a handful of primary lab tests that specifically assess the permeability of the gut lining. Some of these include:

- Cyrex Array 2 Antigenic Permeability Screen

- Genova's Intestinal Permeability Assay
- Zonulin Protein Test

The Cyrex Array 2 Antigenic Permeability Screen is an autoimmune-response test, indicating if the body has inflammatory response pathways and antibodies, commonly associated with the autoimmune attack of leaky gut.

Genova's Intestinal Permeability Assay is a lactulose-mannitol test, which measures levels of these two sugars in your urine after you consume them orally. Since lactulose is naturally a LARGER substance (and should NOT easily end up in your urine), if it does on the test, leaky gut is suspected.

Lastly, a zonulin serum blood test such as the Doctor's Data or GI Map Zonulin Test can also point you in the right direction towards diagnosis.

A key marker of "leaky" gut is **decreased** zonulin levels—an essential protein found in the gut lining that helps keep it nice and strong. Hence, if zonulin is low or out of range, then leaky gut is suspected. The good news? Low zonulin is reversible. In other words: if you discover you have low zonulin, you're able to increase zonulin and CAN improve leaky gut and heal.

What to do about it?

Unlike a missing limb or your brown eyes, you are not bound or stuck with leaky gut forever.

If you suspect you have a leaky gut, the best way to address it head on is to implement the healthy dietary, lifestyle and supplemental gut-healing protocols in this gut kickstart to see if the symptoms resolve on their own.

In addition, while leaky gut testing can be helpful to confirm a diagnosis, it is not always necessary—especially before considering and addressing the other underlying gut pathologies or conditions which may have caused your leaky gut in the first place. **In fact**, there are many other contributing gut issues which will not get picked up on a leaky gut lab test alone.

CHAPTER 5

Beyond Leaky Gut: 8 Reasons Why Your Gut is Imbalanced

Beyond Leaky Gut

A common misconception of poor gut health is that you have a "leaky gut."

However, this is NOT the case for all people. Often, "leaky gut" itself is a byproduct or side effect, not the primary cause, of an unhealthy gut triggered by something else.

In short, even though an estimated three in four Americans alone have "some sort of GI dysfunction" (again, not all have gut-related symptoms), no two *unhealthy* guts are alike, and poor gut health goes far beyond leaky gut.

Eight other common "under the hood" imbalances which can cause an unhealthy gut or leaky gut symptoms include:

1. Low Stomach Acid
2. Food Intolerances
3. SIBO
4. Infections
5. Disrupted Gut Bacteria
6. Toxic Burden
7. Structural Imbalances

8. Lack of "Gut Love"

We won't get too scientific, but let's briefly raise awareness to what these eight gut imbalances look (and feel like) and understand why you may be experiencing poor health (like a slow metabolism, autoimmune disease, acne, allergies, bloating, constipation, and "leaky gut" in the first place).

Knowledge is power.

When we are more aware of what we are feeling—and the underlying gut conditions— we can begin learning more about how to heal for ourselves.

Let's go deeper into those eight other imbalances which can cause an unhealthy gut or leaky gut symptoms.

1. Low Stomach Acid

Stomach acid is good for you. It's necessary to break down food, absorb nutrients, and protect against pathogens. If we're low on it, then *everything else down the digestive tract line* gets thrown off.

As previously discussed, PPIs (proton pump inhibitors) are some of the top-selling drugs of modern day—with more than 15 million Americans trying to suppress their own stomach acid, thinking that it's causing their GERD and heartburn symptoms.

The reality?

Low stomach acid, or "hypochlorhydria," is actually the real cause of GERD and heartburn. When you don't have *enough* stomach acid to digest your food, then of course your food will want to come back up.

Low stomach acid is one of the primary reasons why your gut may be "unhealthy" and is often linked to most of the other pathologies as well. All stressors we've discussed are threats to stomach acid including:

- Antibiotic, NSAID & medication use
- Poor quality foods
- Not chewing your food or slowing down at meals
- Overtraining and too frequent exercise
- Not getting enough sleep
- Underlying infections (H. pylori/fungal)
- Gastritis (inflammation of the stomach lining)
- Pernicious anemia (low Vitamin B12 and loss of parietal cells—stomach lining cells)
- Impaired production of digestive enzymes (carbohydrate, protein or fat malabsorption)
- And other sources of stress

Low stomach acid is a leading cause of a vast majority of lingering gut issues, and is linked to bacterial overgrowth, GERD/heartburn, constipation, bloating, gas, nutrient deficiencies, belching and gas, adult acne and skin breakouts, neurological, blood sugar and hormone imbalances, sleepiness, (especially after meals), headaches, undigested food in stools, IBS, stomach pains or cramps, autoimmune disease, joint pain, loss of taste for meat, and bad breath.

How do I know if I have low stomach acid?

Diagnosis of low stomach acid is not concrete. In a clinic or lab, doctors may use the Heidelberg radiotelemetry test, however given it requires special equipment, many do not use it. The next best method? Self-experimentation. Evaluate your symptoms, such as protein or carbohydrate malabsorption, fullness in the stomach, gas, bloating after meals, and signs of indigestion (GERD). You may also consider doing an "HCL challenge," where you take hydrochloric acid supplements (mimicking stomach acid), and gradually increase the dose until you feel a burning sensation. You would then reduce the dose to the dose you were at just before that burning sensation, and take your HCL with meals. If symptoms improve or lessen, low stomach acid is more than likely warranted.

Gut Love Action

Low stomach acid support or "treatment" includes:

1. Taking an HCL* (hydrochloric acid) tablet with protein-based meals or drinking a tablespoon of apple cider vinegar in water before meals. [*Do not take if currently taking a PPI, corticosteroids or NSAIDs, or pregnant.]
2. If you're taking PPI acid-suppressing drugs, work with your practitioner to transition off those.
3. Replacing and stimulating bile and digestive enzyme production with supplemental Ox Bile and Digestive Enzymes (See "Cheat Sheets" in Resources for recommendations).
4. Possibly try a low-FODMAP diet to see if symptoms don't improve with HCL/Apple Cider Vinegar and enzymes alone.

2. Food Intolerances

Gut problems (like bacterial overgrowth, low stomach acid, gut infections, leaky gut) often go hand-in-hand with food intolerances—certain foods that trigger an inflammatory response inside your gut.

The tricky thing?

You may NOT always FEEL food intolerances in your gut.

In fact, common signs of food intolerances include things like skin breakouts, acne, ADD/ADHD, brain fog, headaches, anxiety, joint pain, nutrient deficiencies, hormonal imbalances, and other non-gut-related symptoms.

We can eat foods for years and suffer the "consequences" without ONCE attributing it to the foods we eat.

To make things even more complicated, we OFTEN crave foods **we are intolerant to**. If you find you crave certain foods that don't always make you feel the best (i.e. you get headaches, heart palpitations, bloating, and/or loose stools), but continue to want to eat them anyways, there IS a reason: Hungry bacteria.

Your bad gut bugs LOVE feeding off foods that ferment in your gut and will signal to your body to eat more of them to make them happy.

This is the reason why you may crave that bag of nuts or sugar time and time again—even though you always feel constipated after you eat them, or the reason why you continue to eat sweet potatoes several times per day, even though bloating happens time and time again.

Your gut bugs like them.

Allergies vs. Intolerances
It's important to understand that an intolerance is not the same as an allergy. Food allergies are IgE- mediated, whereas intolerances are IgG- or IgA-mediated.

IgE, IgG and IgA refers to different types of immunoglobulins or "antibodies" which are part of our immune system and are produced in response to things we come in contact with on a daily basis.

Our bodies create antibodies to foreign substances like bacteria and viral cells, but can also respond to foods, dust, dander, and pollen. Antibodies help the body trigger an immune system response to fight against foreign invaders.

However, when we have TOO many antibodies, this can cause either:

1. An immediate allergic reaction (IgE response), such as watery eyes, diarrhea, hives and difficulty breathing; OR

2. A food sensitivity reaction (IgA and IgG response). Food sensitivity reactions are usually more delayed (several hours to days) and encompass a variety of symptoms not always directly connected to gut health, like:
    - Brain fog
    - Headaches
    - Joint pain
    - Blood sugar imbalances (hypo/hyperglycemia)
    - ADD/ADHD
    - Difficulty concentrating
    - Fatigue
    - Intestinal discomfort
    - Rashes & skin breakouts
    - "Slow" metabolism
    - Malabsorption & nutrient deficiencies

Food allergies are most commonly diagnosed in childhood by an allergist using a skin prick, oral testing, blood test or an oral food challenge/test.

Food intolerances or sensitivities, on the other hand, are rarely assessed in conventional medicine practices. Due to their "silent" and less overt symptoms (which look like other diseases and imbalances), food intolerances often go ***undiagnosed***.

Exhibit A: Gluten

For instance, gluten, the protein found in wheat, is one of the most common food intolerances (both Celiac Disease and non-celiac sensitivity). However, most conventional doctors and allergy panels only test for allergies to "alpha gliadin" (Celiac Disease), failing to screen for other forms of gluten sensitivity, including epitopes of gliadin (beta, gamma, omega), glutenin, wheat germ agglutinin (WGA), gluteomorphin, and deamidated gliadin. Hence, people with Non-Celiac Gluten Sensitivity are even more likely than people with Celiac Disease to go undiagnosed. Moreover, while gluten allergy (Celiac Disease) is highly correlated with symptoms like chronic IBS, loose stools, immediate bloating, fatigue and vomiting upon exposure to gluten, gluten sensitivity and intolerance symptoms can include anything from brittle fingernails and acne to lingering anxiety, low energy and migraines.

In addition, beyond gluten allergies and gluten intolerances alone, there are dozens of other "gluten cross-contaminating" foods many people are often intolerant to that will not always show up on a gluten allergy or intolerance testing, including: coffee (instant), soy, dairy, shellfish/seafood, eggs, peanuts, rice, tapioca, quinoa, buckwheat, and chocolate. And, if you have low digestive enzyme production, stomach acid or bacterial overgrowth, your antibodies may also be triggered by other "healthy" foods, like FODMAPS (i.e. onions, sweet fruits, broccoli, Brussels sprouts), nightshades (eggplants, tomatoes, peppers, potatoes), and even proteins (chicken, turkey, seafood) as well.

How do I know if I have food intolerances?

Blood testing, hair testing, and saliva testing are the current standard methods of testing for food intolerances.

Caution: Not all food intolerance tests are created equal.

Since IgG and IgA food intolerance testing have not been standardized yet, different labs use different methods of testing, and often many labs produce false positives or false negatives.

In short, many food allergy testing methods are NOT 'consistent and reproducible,' meaning if the test is run on the same person's blood or saliva multiple times, it will NOT produce the same or similar results within the range of tolerance. If a test is not consistent, then you simply cannot rely on the results.

Avoid These:
ALCAT
MRT
ELISA

ALCAT & MRT Testing 101
ALCAT (antigen leukocyte cellular antibody test) and MRT (mediator release testing) testing, known as "cytotoxicity testing," are two popular food intolerance tests used by many nutritionists and functional medicine providers that lack consistency and reproducibility.

These tests involve placing a drop of the your blood onto a plate that's coated with a liquid or dried food extract for about 10 minutes. The plate is then examined under a microscope every 30 minutes for the next one to two hours. A technician looks for changes in the structure and shape of the white blood cell. If there are changes in the size or the rounding or the inactivity of the cell, or if it dissolves completely, a positive result is reported.

The problem?

For starters, this testing methodology has never been proven. No study or research has ever shown that measuring changes in white blood cell size is related to food intolerances. Secondly, there are several non-food ingredients in the food extracts used in cytotoxic testing which may potentially interfere with actual blood sample extracts, yielding false positives or false negatives.

ELISA Testing 101

ELISA, IgG and IgG4 testing, is another popular food intolerance test that involves testing a person's blood for immunoglobulin G (IgG). In the lab, a technician adds the blood sample to a petri dish containing specific antigens (such as gluten or wheat, milk, eggs, etc.) related to the condition for which you are being tested. If your blood contains antibodies to the antigen, the two will bind together.

Again, this testing method is not valid, primarily because:

1. ELISA testing has not shown consistent and replicable results from sample to sample;

2. Labs do not always test for foods in the form they are consumed in (i.e. raw vs. cooked). Many labs test for the raw versions of foods alone (eggs, chicken, broccoli, etc.), without regard that you actually may eat those foods cooked. Since cooking changes the proteins in foods, your "positive" reactions to raw forms may not be 100% accurate; and,

3. ELISA (IgG & IgG4 testing alone) completely leaves out IgA antibody testing, too. Since IgG antibodies are the MOST common antibodies in your body, they accumulate with

exposure to the same foods. Hence, if you eat A LOT of nuts or A LOT of sweet potatoes, you can cause a presentation of "food sensitivity" to arise, simply because you have LOTS of IgG's in your body. By measuring IgA also, you validate whether or not your "sensitivity" is just due to eating too much of the same foods versus an actual IgA AND IgG food sensitivity response.

So which test should YOU use?!
If you choose to run a food intolerance test, you want one that tests for both IgG and IgA antibodies, as well as the raw and cooked versions of the foods being tested (instead of raw chicken or potato) and that has been clinically validated.

To date, Cyrex Labs (www.cyrexlabs.com) provides the most comprehensive and reliable blood panel testing for food intolerances, testing for both IgG and IgA antibodies in the forms they are most consumed, and these tests have proven reliability in multiple clinical trials. Cyrex has lab panels you can run directly through many functional medicine practitioners, nutritionist, or the lab itself (they provide you with a clinician to review your results).

Nevertheless, beyond standard labs and food intolerance testing, the gold standard for lab testing involves simply a DIY version at home—elimination and reintroduction.

The Gut Kickstart is a cost-effective, built-in testing method which involves cutting back on the MOST gut-inflammatory foods for 28 days ("20 percent foods" to only eat rarely), followed by a reintroduction period of any suspected trigger foods.

The top most inflammatory foods include:
- Grains & Gluten (some white Jasmine rice may be tolerated)

- Egg Whites
- Pork (slowest digesting meat)
- Nuts
- Nightshades (Chili Powder, Paprika, Tomatoes, Peppers, White Potatoes, Eggplant)
- Conventional Dairy & Meat
- Added Sugar & Artificial Sweeteners (other than pure maple syrup)
- Coffee (No more than once per day)
- Chocolate—Less than 80% dark
- Alcohol
- Soy
- Vegetable Oils
- Peanuts & Legumes (some may tolerate beans if soaked and sprouted)
- Processed & GMO Foods (including some gluten-free processed foods; the only thing missing in many of these products is gluten! Some still contain gut inflammatory sugars and oils; use judgment)

In addition, some people are sensitive to FODMAPS like cruciferous veggies (broccoli, Brussels sprouts, cauliflower) and high amounts of fructose (lots of fruit in a day), so it is encouraged that you use your own judgement with these foods.

So what CAN I eat?

Hundreds of foods! Even though inflammatory foods seemingly seem like "all the good" foods, there are hundreds of nourishing foods to eat in abundance. See your Gut Love Nutrition Plan for all the details.

The ultimate purpose?

Not to starve or deprive your body, but to enliven your body and reawaken your true gut intuition in order to assess whether you are intolerant to certain foods or not.

Like a dirty windshield with lots of dirt on it, sometimes we don't realize we are intolerant to foods until we take them out and then reintroduce them. If our windshield is "clean," our body is able to tell us whether or not that food sits with us.

3. SIBO (Small Intestinal Bacterial Overgrowth)

Small intestinal bacterial overgrowth is the build up or "overgrowth" of bacteria in the small intestine. Most commonly it is an overgrowth of various types of bacteria found in the colon. This bacteria travels to the small intestine and sets up camp. It can also result from an increase in the normal bacteria of the small intestine, though this is less common. A healthy gut microbiome consists of only 10,000 bacteria in the sterile small intestine, and about **10 times that amount in the large intestine.**

When the small intestine gets over taxed with too much bacteria, these bacteria may significantly interfere with digestion of food and absorption of nutrients, primarily by damaging the cells lining the small bowel (the mucosa). This damage to the small bowel mucosa can lead to "leaky gut" (when the intestinal barrier becomes permeable, allowing large protein molecules to escape into the bloodstream). These bacteria, whether too many or the wrong types, can also lead to nutritional deficiencies thanks to poor digestion or absorption. Bacteria take up vitamins and amino acids before our own cells have a chance to absorb these nutrients.

Over time, this causes a host of other gut symptoms as well, including:

- Bloating within 1-2 hours of eating and abdominal distension
- Diarrhea
- Passing gas frequently
- Chronic constipation (no matter how much water and fiber you consume) or IBS
- Stomach upset, especially when you eat carbohydrates and sugars
- Brittle nails
- Acne and skin breakouts
- Blood sugar imbalances (i.e. hungry every 2-3 hours, hypo/hyperglycemic episodes, insatiable cravings for sugar or caffeine)
- Inflammation (like high cholesterol)
- Weight gain or weight loss
- Food intolerances
- Migraines and chronic headaches
- ADD/ADHD and brain fog

Sound familiar?

Remember, the gut is the gateway to health and bloating and constipation are not the only signs that something is "up" in your gut.

The three primary causes of Small Intestinal Bacterial Overgrowth include:

1. Low stomach acid
2. Dysfunction of gut motility (ie. impaired ability of organs to push food through the gut)
3. Disrupted gut bacteria, particularly in the large intestine (from poor quality foods, undigested foods, prior food poisoning, antibiotics, toxic burden and lifestyle stressors)

How do I know if I have SIBO?

The two primary methods currently used to diagnose SIBO are SIBO breath testing and the aspiration of the small bowel using an endoscope. Since endoscopy is expensive and uncomfortable, the SIBO breath test is the most popular and preferred test of choice.

It involves breathing into a sample collection tube and bag at home every 20 minutes over the course of 3 hours.

One to two days before the test, you are also advised to cut out all high-fiber and lactose-containing foods, including a vegetables, all fruits, all nuts and seeds (and nut milks), all beans, all grains (except limited white rice), all condiments, and all spices and herbs (except salt and pepper). These foods contain sugars that bacteria love. Limiting starches and sugars in foods prior to the test allows results to fully showcase whether or not you naturally have MORE bacteria in the gut. Acceptable foods to eat one to two days prior to the test include: meat, fish, seafood, poultry, plain steamed white rice, meat broth, fats and oils (coconut oil, ghee), eggs, salt and pepper, and organic weak black coffee or black tea.

During the test, hydrogen and methane gases are collected for assessment. Since SIBO is associated with an OVERPRODUCTION of either or both of these gases, test results will indicate if your body has increased levels when you breathe into the test tube.

That said, false positives are not abnormal. Lab testing is not perfect and if results come back "negative," SIBO is not always ruled out. In fact, "silent SIBO" (a.k.a. "Hydrogen-Sulfide" SIBO) is often supposed if SIBO test results come back nearly at "0," with seemingly no measure of hydrogen or methane based gas at all, and if gut symptoms and SIBO-related symptoms still persist. Hydrogen-Sulfide SIBO is not evaluated during standard breath testing and should not be ruled out, and a 30-60 day SIBO antimicrobial treatment and dietary protocol may still be warranted.

Is there another way to tell aside from testing?
If lab testing is not in the cards for you, it is a commonly accepted belief that if your clinical signs indicate you may have SIBO, a short-term treatment trial using a SIBO gut-healing protocol is *better* than not treating for SIBO at all.

SIBO treatment typically consists of an anti-inflammatory diet (ie. this gut kickstart) coupled with a targeted, antimicrobial (herbal) supplement and gut-healing protocol (probiotics, prebiotics, enzymes, etc.).

The thought behind this theory is that: **IF SIBO is present, then the targeted SIBO healing protocol will do more good than harm.** And if SIBO is NOT present, then the only real "consequence" is that SIBO treatment won't work for you (because you may have not had SIBO in the first place, but something else—like a viral or parasitic infection, low stomach acid, etc.)

Many functional medicine practitioners and nutritionists are familiar with SIBO testing and the best people to connect with for official diagnosis. (See your Cheat Sheet SIBO Protocol in the Resources for more information).

4. Infections (Parasitic & Bacterial)

Parasites

A **parasite** is any organism that lives and feeds off of another organism. When we talk about gut **parasites**, imagine tiny organisms like worms, which feed off of your body and nutrition.

There are hundreds of different parasites with long names that are difficult to pronounce including: cryptosporidium ("crypto"), Blastocystis hominis ("blasto"); Dientamoeba fragilis; Giardia lamblia; Entamoeba histolytica, or e-histolytica; ascaris; Necator americanus, (hookworm); Enterobius vermicularis (pinworm); Entamoeba coli; and Entamoeba hartmanni. (Try saying any one of those seven times fast!).

Parasitic infections are caused by:

- Ingesting poor quality or uncooked foods (i.e. food poisoning or infection from water in Mexico)
- Sanitation (not washing your hands, or dirty water)
- Contamination from animals (i.e. feces in natural water streams or exposure to contaminants from pets)
- Contamination at daycare centers
- Antibiotic use
- Insect bites
- Other toxic exposures.

Moreover, just ONE bad run of food poisoning or ONE trip overseas, drinking or ingesting a bad source of water, is powerful enough to give you a parasitic infection that may linger for years.

In fact, parasites can hang around in many folks for 10 or more years (or longer) before any diagnosis, especially since the symptoms of parasitic, fungal or bacterial infection may sound similar to *other* gut-symptoms and health woes we've already discussed, including: bloating, IBS, diarrhea, and constipation, to fatigue, brain fog, memory loss, insomnia, skin breakouts, hormonal imbalances and inflammatory chronic diseases (high cholesterol, autoimmune conditions, heart disease, diabetes, etc.).

Once again, a vast majority of people don't even report gut symptoms at all. (Shocker!)

Parasitic infections cause these conditions by invading gut cells, damaging the intestines and gut barrier lining, and further weakening the immune system. (Remember, the gut is the gateway to health, and 80% of your immune cells alone are in your gut). The body's defense mechanisms decline and welcome in body breakdown.

Common Parasites:
- Giardia
- Cryptosporidium
- Entamoeba coli
- Blastocystis species (most common parasite in the U.S.)
- Dientamoeba fragilis

Bacterial Infections

Similar to parasites, bacterial infections are also difficult to detect and know if you have them or not, primarily due to the broad range of health symptoms, not always associated with the gut.

Common names of bacteria that can cause gut infections include: Clostridium, H. pylori, Escherichia coli, Bacillus, "Staph," and Salmonella.

Not ALL bacteria are bad, but the overgrowth of bacteria—particularly "pathogenic" (disease-causing) bacteria"—is where health problems arise.

Bacterial infection can occur through similar means as parasites and other gut pathologies, including:

- Food poisoning
- Medicines
- Contamination (water, pet, sexual)
- Toxins in cleaning, beauty and hygiene supplies, and environment

- Poor quality foods (processed, packaged, hydrogenated oils, artificial sweeteners, etc.)

A high amount or acute (sudden) exposure to pathogenic bacteria, such as salmonella in uncooked chicken, can trigger infection in the gut.

How do I know if I have parasitic or bacterial infection?:

A comprehensive stool test is the best way to confirm what—if any—parasites or pathogenic bacteria are at play.

It is recommended you run a "Comprehensive Stool Analysis," which has the capability to identify more than 1000 different bacteria and fungal organisms, such as the Doctor's Data Comprehensive Stool Analysis or Biohealth 401H. These tests typically also assess at least three samples' worth of stool, since parasitic infections are notorious for hiding in the body, and often go undetected on just one stool sample alone.

Blood testing and organic acids testing also exist. Most conventional doctors and hospital panels use PCR or DNA/PCR based methods, which are great for evaluating if one or two certain organisms (you are already looking for) are in the stool (such as E.Coli or Salmonella from food poisoning), but they do not give a clear overall big picture of all the bacteria that is there like a comprehensive stool analysis does.

A stool test will display what, if any, specific parasites or pathogenic bacteria may be present as well as other inflammatory markers associated with disease, including:

- Lysozyme (gut inflammation)
- Lactoferrin (marker for Irritable Bowel Disease)
- Calprotectin (Irritable Bowel Disease)
- Red blood cells &/or mucus in stool

- Fecal elastase or fat stains (greasy stools)
- Secretory IgA (first line of defense against pathogens, so if it is out of range, parasites and infections are more likely)
- Low short chain fatty acid production (short chain fatty acids are produced by healthy bacteria ideally)
- Undigested food in stools (carb or protein malabsorption)

5. Disrupted Gut Bacteria (Dysbiosis)

Our health is governed by our gut bacteria. Your gut is home to trillions of bacteria, both "good" and "bad," and ideally, you want the "Goldilocks" (just right) amount for a balance of each.

When things get out of balance, "dysbiosis" happens.

Dysbiosis may present as:

- Too few good bacteria and too many bad bacteria
- Low production or absence of good bacteria (even if bad bacteria levels are normal)
- Too many of individual strains of bacteria (even if they are good)

Dysbiosis, or bacterial imbalances can lead to side effects like inflammation, bloating, constipation, IBS, leaky gut, nutrient deficiencies, malabsorption and other health imbalances (from chronic headaches to allergies, skin breakouts and anxiety).

Disrupted gut bacteria (dysbiosis) is different from bacterial and parasitic infections, because it simply means there is an IMBALANCE of good and bad bacteria in your gut. Aside from OUTSIDE infection by disease-causing gut bacteria in infections, the simple overgrowth of bacteria or underproduction of good bacteria (which you ALREADY HAVE in your gut) can cause disrupted gut bacteria (dysbiosis) or "fungal overgrowth."

Candida is a prime example of this. You naturally have yeast in your belly—and yeast is not necessarily a bad thing (as long as you don't have too much of it). In the case of Candida, yeast becomes overgrown due to various lifestyle stressors (such as high carbohydrate consumption, a round of antibiotics, birth control pills, artificial sweeteners, etc.) and symptoms similar to SIBO arise, including: bloating and GI issues, depression, anxiety, brain fog, ADHD, autism spectrum disorder, skin issues, and allergies.

How does Dysbiosis happen?

Generally speaking, dysbiosis (bacteria imbalance) happens when bacteria invade the GI tract from the overexposure to poor quality foods, stress, medications; the structure of your gut changes; and/or you lack beneficial probiotics and prebiotics to support a healthy ecosystem.(Hawkrelak & Myers, 2004 http://www.altmedrev.com/publications/9/2/180.pdf).

In short, too much of any one good thing (bacteria type) is not a good thing. Disrupted gut bacteria arises when you have too much of any one type of bacteria and an imbalance in bacterial strains present.

How do I know if I have "disrupted gut bacteria?"

The same stool tests used to assess parasites and bacterial infections can assess the profile of bacteria in your gut. Organic Acids Testing (a urine test) can also be used as a marker for microbial overgrowth. Additionally, if you ever feel sick when you take probiotics (particularly lactic acid bacteria probiotics) this can be an indicator of bacterial overgrowth or imbalance.

There are four types of bacterial presentations to assess on a stool test:

1. **Expected/beneficial flora.** The "beneficial" bacteria that IDEALLY makes up the majority of total bacteria in a healthy and balanced GI tract. These beneficial bacteria have health-promoting effects like boosted mood, metabolism, hormones, skin health and immune function.

2. **Clostridia** These are also prevalent bacteria in a healthy intestine. However, if Clostridium species' are low or overgrown, dysbiosis can still happen.

3. **Commensal (imbalanced) flora.** Neither pathogenic nor beneficial to your host GI tract. However, if there are low levels of beneficial bacteria and increased levels of commensal bacteria, imbalances may occur.

4. **Dysbiotic flora.** Also known as "pathogenic" or "bad" bacteria, since they have the potential to cause disease and inflammation in the GI tract. Some popular strain names include: Klebsiella, Citrobacter freundii, H. pylori (some may be beneficial, but mostly known as pathogenic).

What do I do about it?

Treatment of dysbiosis usually includes a combination of spore-based probiotics, combined with easily-digestible prebiotics (like partially hydrolyzed guar gum) and potentially a short-term low FODMAP (low sugar/starch) diet to see if symptoms improve. In addition, prebiotic- and probiotic-rich foods can help. (See your Gut Kickstart Nutrition Plan later on in this book for more info).

6. Toxic Burden (Liver/Gallbladder Dysfunction)

Your liver is your primary "detoxifying" organ—the filtration system in your body that decides what foods, toxins, chemicals and substances you ingest, inhale or come into contact with (hygiene products, cleaning products, environments, plastics, etc.) stay inside or go back out into your body.

It's like the master garbage disposal and recycling machine—all in one.

Unfortunately, the liver goes "awry" (like the rest of your gut health) when it is stressed—leaving it to function less than optimally, unable to remove toxins out of your body appropriately (often leaving unwanted toxins in your body and leading to digestive stress).

Common reasons why your liver gets overworked or stressed include:

- NSAIDs, birth control pills, and long-term prescription medication use
- Frequent alcohol consumption
- Processed foods & hydrogenated oils (eating out a lot)
- Sedentary lifestyles or overtraining
- Pesticides in your fruits and veggies
- Conventionally raised meats and dairy
- Processed diet foods with dyes, chemicals, and artificial sweeteners
- Heavy metal exposure (farmed fish, dental work, surgical procedures)
- Mold exposure (apartment, home)
- Plastic container and plastic water bottle use
- Electromagnetic radiation

- Contaminated water
- Toxic cleaning supplies, beauty supplies and hygiene products
- Nail polish, hairspray and perfume fumes
- Gasoline inhalation

We are exposed to thousands of environmental toxins every day. In fact, the average woman uses 120 chemicals in her beauty products in the morning alone. (Fun Fact: The skin is the largest organ in your body—what you put onto your skin is absorbed directly into your body. If you would not eat it, don't use it on your skin).

Signs of liver toxicity or toxic overload may look like:
- Difficulty digesting fat—even healthy fat
- Stubborn belly fat, rolls or a "pot belly"
- Dark circles under your eyes
- Elevated LDL cholesterol, reduced HDL cholesterol, and elevated triglycerides
- Overheating of the body or excessive perspiration
- Gallbladder removal or attacks
- Pain or discomfort in right upper abdominal area under the rib cage
- Skin breakouts, dry skin, or blotchy skin
- Chronic fatigue
- Light or clay colored stools
- Frequent nausea
- Greasy or shiny stools
- Easily intoxicated or sick if you drink wine
- Bitter taste in mouth (especially after meals)
- Motion sickness
- Cravings for sugar
- Foggy brain

- Bad breath
- Hypoglycemia
- Pain between shoulder blades
- Sensitive to chemicals and smells
- Elevated AST or ALT levels on routine blood work
- Toxic metal overload (assessed typically by a hair test)
- Unexplained weight gain, or inability to lose weight (even with "clean eating")
- Estrogen dominance (80% of women over the age of 35 have estrogen dominance–and desperately need the periodic liver optimization).

Although we CAN'T live in a bubble, there are measures we can take in our daily lives to support our liver and make sure it is detoxifying appropriately—including the steps you'll learn in this gut kickstart, with special mindfulness not only to the foods we eat and supplements we take, but also to the beauty, cleaning, and hygiene products we use, electronics attached to our hip, food storage containers, water sources, and more.

How do I know if I have liver toxicity?

Blood testing can be one indicator of liver toxicity—specifically:

- **High AST** (Aspartate aminotransferase): normal is between 0-23 IU/L for women and 0-25 IU/L for men
- **High ALT** (Alanine aminotransferase) normal is between 0-20 for women, and 0-26 for men
- **GGT:** normal is 0-21 IU/L for women, 0-29 IU/L for men
- **LDH:** normal is 140-180 IU/L
- **Alkaline phosphatase:** normal is 42-107 IU/L, and/or:
- **Low creatinine:** normal is 0.7-1.0 mg/dL for women, 0.85-1.1 mg/dL for men

Hair testing and urine testing are also laboratory methods for clinical assessment of toxic burden—revealing certain metals, molds, or toxic exposures.

7. Structural Imbalances

Still feel badly or experience GI symptoms despite treating or addressing pathogenic imbalances and stressors (bacteria, parasites, fungus, leaky gut)?

Beyond these top disease-driven pathogens, if things are still not "getting better," there may be justification to look at what is going on structurally in your GI tract.

Blockage, obstructions and chronic inflammation of your intestines are other less common and less discussed considerations, yet equally important if you've exhausted other possibilities of gut imbalances.Aside from the pathologies we've discussed to assess first, common "outlier" GI conditions include:

Diverticulitis. This is a disease which affects the large intestine, characterized by inflammation due to small bulges or pockets (diverticula) in the lining of the intestine. These bulges get there in the first place primarily due to inflammation from the processed foods you ate as a kid, poor eating hygiene (not chewing your food, etc.), a leaky gut and low stomach acid, chronic stress (poor sleep, psychological stress, working out too much or not enough, etc.), and more. Fecal calprotectin (a **measurement of the protein calprotectin in your stool**) can be assessed to identify intestinal inflammation, and is reported to be higher in those with diverticular disease (Tursi, 2014).

The most common symptoms include lower abdominal pain, bloating, diarrhea or abdominal pain (particularly on the left side), however a large majority of individuals affected by diverticulitis do not present with symptoms at all. It is estimated that one in two people will develop diverticula by the time they are 80 years old. Surgery for diverticulitis to remove bulges is rare, and the most common line of defense entails reducing intestinal inflammation by doing what you've learned to do thus far: Balancing your gut bacteria, continuing to support the gut via a real-foods lifestyle and plenty of carbohydrates (fibrous and some real-food starches), and improving intestinal motility (below) to prevent diverticulitis attacks.

Megacolon (Enlarged Bowel). Megacolon is the term used for an abnormally enlarged colon. It is often associated with extra (redundant) loops of bowel. It can cause severe constipation. Megacolon is a structural and mechanical issue and can trigger abdominal bloating, constipation, flatulence and pain. While many people turn to enemas, coffee enemas, colonics, laxatives, fiber or probiotics to help relieve chronic constipation and bloating, in the case of a megacolon, this is not completely solved with strong herbs, colonic irrigations, or supplements alone. In fact, in some with severe constipation caused by a megacolon, there is damage to the nerves that supply the muscles in the colon, making the contractions of the muscles become weaker and preventing the feces from moving along the colon. Diagnosis of a megacolon is made via a special X-ray called a barium enema, revealing the extra loops of unwanted bowel. If a megacolon is found, extreme cases may warrant surgery (bowel resection) to remove the extra loops of bowel and rejoin the healthy edges of the colon. The symptoms are relieved and the constipation cured. This surgical procedure is called a bowel resection and is best done by a surgeon who specializes in large bowel (colon) surgery. Surgery is only warranted after lifestyle measures have first been taken to optimize bowel health, including:

- **Enough Water + Balanced Real-Food Diet** with plenty of healthy fats and fiber leafy greens. In addition, a fiber support supplement can be beneficial.
- **Prebiotics + Probiotics**
- **Stress Management**
- **Liver support with herbs and supplements.** Your liver makes bile, which is a natural laxative for your body. If your liver isn't keeping up with the job, you can expect your bowel function to slow down. Common herbs and supplements for liver support include: Ox bile, cod liver oil, Taurine supplementation, dandelion root, milk thistle, Turmeric, barberry, and globe artichoke, along with eating beets, organ meats, raw vegetable juice and potassium-rich foods like sweet potatoes, bananas, blackstrap molasses, and spinach.

Intestinal Obstruction. Intestinal obstruction is characterized like many other "gut issues" (constipation, chronic abdominal pain, loss of appetite, inability to have a bowel movement or pass gas, and/or abdominal swelling). Essentially it is exactly what it sounds like—an obstruction or blockage somewhere in the intestinal tract, most commonly linked to former pelvic or abdominal surgery or colon cancer. However, other common causes include: Hernias, which are portions of intestine that protrude into another part of your body, IBD (inflammatory bowel disease), diverticulitis, twisting of the colon or impacted feces.

There are several tests your practitioner will run if intestinal obstruction is suspected including physical exam, an abdominal X-Ray (however, not all intestinal obstructions can be detected on X-ray), a CT scan (generally more accurate), and/or an air or barium enema (aka "colon X-ray"). To conduct an air or barium enema, the doctor will insert air or liquid barium into the colon through an enema in the rectum and view an enhanced image of the colon on an X-ray. Depending on findings, treatment varies from dietary and lifestyle changes alone to surgery if complete blockage is suspected. If the cause of your intestinal obstruction is due to an underlying pathology (i.e. IBD, fungal or bacterial overgrowth), then continued healing and treatment of those underlying pathologies is warranted, with plenty of gut-healing and soothing interventions, as well. Most GI docs will typically recommend a "lower fiber diet" that they say is "easier for your bowel to process," but we know about the role of prebiotics (fiber) along with probiotics, cooked vegetables (particularly leafy greens), and other intestinal-healing foods, supplements and herbs (bone broth, fermented yogurt, glutamine, aloe vera, slippery elm, licorice, and turmeric/curcumin), and these are a good first-line of defense.

Slowed Colon Motility. Simply put: Not going (as much) or frequent constipation. There can be multiple reasons for a "slower bowel motility" (pooping time), but a common reason amongst many is low serotonin. For this reason, slowed colon motility is common in individuals who struggle with anxiety, depression, and other mental illnesses, as serotonin (your "feel-good" brain chemical) is also low in these people. What to do about it? For some, this simply means supplementation with 5-HTP (a precursor to serotonin) to help alleviate alleviate constipation and increase motility since it will increase serotonin levels; however, if the individual is on an SSRI medication, this is not advised without first talking to your doctor. Other treatments for slowed colon motility include ensuring you are eating *enough* starchy (real food) tubers and prebiotic foods, like sweet potatoes, plantains, winter squash, onions, jicama, taro, beets, pumpkin and carrots. In addition, magnesium supplementation can be beneficial for relaxing your intestinal muscles and alleviating constipation.

Colon Cancer. Lastly, colon and rectum cancer is the second leading cause of cancer death in the United States. However, colon cancer is typically referred to as "one of the most preventable" due to the influence of dietary choices and overall GI health. Cancer itself is a symptom—**not** a pathology (underlying cause of symptoms), and even if you are genetically predispositioned for colon cancer, by addressing the lifestyle factors and underlying causes we've discussed thus far (SIBO, fungi, dysbiosis, etc.), you arm your gut with "steel armor" (making it less susceptible to disease).

> **Myth Buster:** *Red meat and protein does not cause cancer. A leaky gut and poor quality foods—including most conventional meat—carcinogens, toxins, pesticides, sugar and hydrogenated oils does cause cancer. Opt for sustainably raised, grass-fed and organic meats as much as possible.*

Gut Kickstart Insider Tip

Do I Need a Colonoscopy or upper gastrointestinal (GI) endoscopy?!

If you see a traditional GI doctor first for your gut "problems," sometimes that practitioner will recommend a colonoscopy or endoscopy to see what's going on "under the hood"—particularly if irregularities are found on an X-Ray or CT scan or abdominal pain persists.

A scope of both the colon and upper GI is a more invasive procedure in which a doctor uses an endoscope—a long, flexible tube with a camera—to see the lining of your upper GI tract (the esophagus, stomach, and first part of the small intestine - the duodenum) or lower GI tract (colon) to assess for "unexplained" symptoms including heartburn, abdominal pain, IBS,

> *problems swallowing, unexplained weight loss, GI bleeding, nausea and diarrhea.*
>
> *However, remember, knowing what you know now about overall gut health, rarely should this be the first line of a defense before lifestyle factors and other testing is assessed (i.e. SIBO, fungal and parasitic overgrowth, food intolerances, stress, etc.).*
>
> *Colonoscopies and endoscopies are best used for diagnosing and assessing structural abnormalities (such as intestinal blockage), IBD (Crohn's or Ulcerative Colitis) and inflammation of the GI.*
>
> *While complications with a scope are traditionally said to be rare and minor, one of the most pertinent risks associated with the procedure is irritation of the gut lining—which may trigger more inflammation.*
>
> *Perforation — poking a hole in the intestine — only occurs in 1 in 1000 procedures, but individuals more often risk infection of the colon with unsterilized scope equipment or infection by one of the common sterilizers (glutaraldehyde) itself, which is actually shown to cause colitis **after** the scope is performed (Hsiang-Yao Shih et al, 2011).*

8. Lack of "Loving Your Gut"

Last but not least, what is the #1 underlying factor of all gut dysfunction?

Lack of gut love—mentally, physically and/or emotionally.

In short, stress—the MOST common theme amongst every single "gut issue."

"Lack of gut love" looks different for all people, and can include, but is not limited to:

- Binge eating and disordered eating habits
- Negative self-talk
- Excessive worry over food, body and exercise
- Overthinking and overanalyzing your health
- Anxiety controlling your thoughts
- Burning a candle at both ends and lack of sleep
- Running on caffeine
- High sugar or processed food consumption
- Sedentary lifestyles
- Circadian rhythm dysfunction

Essentially anything that disconnects us from our core—our gut—and stresses us (and/or our physical bodies) out and thwarts cortisol (our stress hormones), without the ability to adequately recover from that stress.

The body (and gut) desire balance. When things get out of sorts, our digestive wellness (and consequently the rest of our wellness) is the first to go.

It's been estimated that upwards of 90% of ALL illnesses and visits to the ER and doctor are for "stress-related pathologies"—physically and/or mentally (AIS, 2017).

Considering this, how do you think your own stress levels and thought patterns are contributing to your personal health and gut health—or lack thereof?

The tricky thing: Often, our daily lifestyle stressors, self-talk, negative thoughts and worries become our "norm" and we STOP considering them to be stressors at all. Which is exactly why I call "stress" the "pink elephant in the room" when it comes to "healing your gut." Are you dancing with pink elephants?

Stress stinks. Loving our gut entails addressing the elephant in the room—and kicking it to the curb.

CHAPTER 6

Dancing with Pink Elephants: Addressing Stress

Stress and disease and gut problems go hand-in-hand—which totally makes sense, considering:

- 80 percent of your immune system and inflammatory-fighting cells are produced in your gut
- 90 percent of your serotonin (feel-good brain chemicals) is made in your gut
- You have MORE neurons (nerve cells that transmit information to and from the brain) in your gut than any other system of your body
- 31 hormones are produced in your gut
- We have 10 times the amount of gut bacteria cells than we do human cells, and the health (or unhealthiness) of your gut bacteria is linked to diseases such as: cancer, Alzheimer's, mood and brain function, allergies, metabolism, hormone and thyroid imbalances, and other inflammatory conditions.

In short, if your body is stressed, then your gut gets stressed and you become sick, unhealthy or experience a number of "signs and symptoms" that technically are not "normal."

Just because symptoms like bloating, constipation, gas after meals, acne, allergies, high blood pressure, high cholesterol, hypothyroidism, needing coffee to function, sugar cravings and hormone imbalances are "normal" in our society doesn't mean these are actually the optimal way your body was designed or wired to live and survive.

Understanding the Link Between the Gut & Stress

Unfortunately, stress gets easily overlooked in our rat-race modern day society.

Especially since bumper-to-bumper rush hour traffic, Roundup pesticide spray on our apples, sulfates in our shampoo, 6-8 hours daily spent staring at screens, and completely booked schedules are ALSO considered "normal".

Consequently, stress takes the form of the "pink elephant in the room." We know it's there. It sticks out and makes us feel unwell, but there's really no escaping it, it's not going anywhere. So we stop paying attention. We learn to deal with it, function, and *survive* (as best as we can).

Humans are innately wired for survival, and our gut is wired to help us survive, too. Although we no longer live in the great outdoors, where tigers, bears and lions roamed freely and natural disasters or life-or-death-survival was the #1 stressor of most humans, our steady influx of modern-day stressors are equally (or arguably more) stressful than the days of old.

Your gut fights to keep stress at bay.

Interestingly, one of the key roles of your gut bacteria is sending signals to your brain in order to cope with elevated "stressors."

In the midst of deadlines, rush hour, takeout pizza, artificial sweeteners, long-term low-carb diets, less than six hours of sleep, blue light screen exposure, and Advil popping, our bodies (and gut bacteria) are **constantly on high alert—often subconsciously sending out a "stress response" signals all day long.**

A normal "stress response" of the body (i.e. the "fight or flight" response) can involve reactions such as:

Physiological
- Increased blood sugar levels
- Increased heart rate and blood pressure to prepare for action
- Dilated pupils
- Constricted veins in the skin to send more blood to major muscle groups (and colder hands and feet)
- Suppressed digestion
- Shortness of breath
- Rapid breathing
- Sweating
- Headaches
- Tense muscles

Psychological
- Constantly thinking about the stressor
- Worry
- Apprehension
- Anxiety
- Difficulty concentrating
- Mood swings
- Assumptions

Your gut bacteria sends these response signals to your brain when you're stressed.

In the case of chronic (ongoing) stress—like poor gut health—even though you may not experience rapid breathing, dilated pupils or tense muscles, if your body is *constantly* stressed, the **internal mechanisms** which govern the stress response (i.e. cortisol, your "stress hormone") are **completely thrown out of whack.**

It's like your body is running from a bear at all times.

Enter: Disease, inflammation and gut problems!

Stress is NOT Just Mental
Many people just think about stress as "mental stress."

However, **mental stress is not solely responsible** for contributing to the "gut-stress conundrum." Physical stressors also play a role.

You could be sitting on a beach in Tahiti, no care or worry in the world, but your body still be stressed: Suffering from SIBO, eczema, allergies and blood sugar dips—relying on coffee or sugar to function.

Address (All Types of) Stress=Heal the Gut
Let's take a peek at 20 of the most common everyday stressors potentially wreaking havoc on your gut health, which we will take care of through your 28-day reset protocol. Warning: these go beyond saying "om" or deep breathing.

See if any of these are issues you have and learn how to address them:

1. Eating poor quality food (GMO, pesticides, antibiotic and grain-fed meat, packaged, processed, conventional dairy, etc.)

2. Eating foods you are intolerant to
3. Chronic under-eating
4. Eating too few carbs
5. Sugar & artificial sweetener consumptions
6. Practicing poor food hygiene (not washing your hands prior to eating, not chewing your food well, eating on the go, eating mindlessly, consuming older or expired foods, etc.)
7. Vitamin P deficiency (lack of pleasure in eating)
8. High coffee consumption
9. High screen exposure and LED blue light
10. Overtraining or sedentary lifestyle
11. Lack of time in nature and fresh air
12. Social media overload
13. Lack of meaningful relationships and community
14. Environmental toxin exposure (ie. plastics, hygiene products, cleaning supplies, etc.)
15. Antibiotic history
16. Life stressors (work, traffic, relationships, etc.)
17. Burning a candle at both ends
18. Disruptions in gut health impacting brain health
19. Not listening to your body, your head or your heart
20. Low self-esteem

The Bottom Line
You cannot heal or address your gut health without first addressing stress, and stress reduction + gut healing go hand in hand, at the same time

The Stress-Gut Connection: 20 Common Stressors that Wreak Havoc on Your Gut

1. Food Quality

Food matters—especially for your gut health.

Like your heart or brain, your digestive system is *constantly working* to process and break down the foods you eat, deliver nutrients, filter toxins, and govern your metabolic processes.

Long after you've finished your morning scramble or lunchtime chicken salad, each meal takes 24 to 72 hours to move through your digestive tract. During sleep your gut also is working—detoxifying, repairing gut cells in your intestinal wall, and sending out vitamins and minerals to restore and repair tissues, organs, bones, hormones and cells.

That said, the quality of the foods we choose to eat can be nourishing or stressful for our gut and overall health. Unfortunately, a vast majority of society does not think about food beyond what it tastes like or how many calories, carbs or fats are in it. But food goes beyond lighting up our taste buds or staying within a predetermined calorie count. While food most certainly is meant to be pleasurable, it is also "fuel."

Consider a plant and a Ferrari.

What does a plant need to survive and thrive? Water, sunshine and rich soil, right?
How about a Ferrari? Premium gasoline, right?

What would happen if you poured gas on a plant? It would die. And what would happen if you put water into the gas tank of a Ferrari? It wouldn't go and would ruin the car.

Your body and gut works the same way. It is innately designed to need and thrive upon a balance of certain foods—proteins, carbohydrates (especially vegetables), healthy fats and water. And not just a balance of these foods—but the true, real deal, best quality sources of these foods.

It doesn't take a rocket scientist to recognize the difference between a 99-cent conventional egg from a chicken raised inhumanely and administered antibiotics and hormones to grow faster, versus an egg from a chicken raised in his natural environment on a real-food diet in a free-roaming pasture. The same thing goes for the apple that grew on the farm or orchard near town, versus the apple shipped in on a hot truck from Mexico two weeks ago. Or beef and dairy from a cow that ate a grain-based diet versus the cow that ate grass on a farm.

How is the *quality* of your food the majority of the time?

No, food perfection is not expected—or possible (We *can't* live in bubbles).

But you do get a choice on what you "invest" into your health savings account every day through the quality of foods you eat within an 80/20 balanced perspective. (Note: Hyper-obsession and stress over eating perfectly is a whole other stressor we will talk about later that equally diminishes your gut health—Vitamin P Deficiency).

2. Healthy Food That Hurts

Although there are hundreds of different food philosophies and diets out there, most people can agree that "healthy" eating entails eating more fresh foods than packaged, processed or sugar-rich ones. However, beyond "fresh foods," what do you do when you are eating "all the right healthy things," BUT your digestion is still off? No matter how many green salads, nuts, eggs, or sweet potatoes you eat, you STILL have digestive symptoms!

I call this conundrum: "Healthy Food That Hurts."

A common (gut health) stressor that health and wellness-minded folks run into is eating foods we've been told or heard are "clean," BUT not being able to digest them. While that broccoli, sweet potato, apple with almond butter, or grilled salmon may be healthy, they may NOT be healthy for your body RIGHT NOW.

I've been there, got the t-shirt.

After 15 years spent fighting my body and following hundreds of food rules in my eating disorder, by the time I was 24, I was over the diet war.

However, while I definitely had more peace with food, I found myself in an entirely new war with my body (or rather, felt like my body was at war with me).

Not in an "I-hate-my-body" type of way, but in a, **"I am scared of what my body will do if I eat this"** sort of way.

Although I was eating "healthy food" and doing everything "right" in my recovery…why did I still *feel so lousy inside?*

- Nuts had me curled in a ball on the floor, wondering why shooting sharp pains struck.
- Eggs made me feel queasy all morning long.
- Sweet potatoes left me in the bathroom several times throughout the day.
- Bison never settled.
- I liked the idea of adding goat cheese to a salad, or eating a homemade paleo almond butter cookie, but my constipation would last for days if I did.

"What gives?!" I wondered—frustrated with why eating foods (that I finally made peace with) hurt so much.

The answer?

My gut. Thanks to **SEVERAL** imbalances in my own gut and health after my previous (stressful) 15 years spent mistreating my body, my body was not 100 percent happy, and it often experienced gas, bloating, loose stools, constipation and unexplained stomach pains when I ate to prove it.

The same thing goes for you. You may be doing everything right on paper and eating "all the right things," but the biggest indicator of what is healthy for your body RIGHT NOW goes back to asking your gut, "How do you feel?"

Common "trigger" or inflammatory "healthy" foods include:

- Nuts and seeds
- Egg whites
- Pork
- Dairy (cheese, milk, yogurt, whey)
- Conventionally-raised meats
- FODMAP foods (apples, broccoli, brussels sprouts, cauliflower, mango, peaches, etc.)
- Nightshades (tomatoes, white potatoes, eggplant, chili powder, bell pepper)
- Grains
- Beans and peanuts
- Soy
- Natural and artificial sweeteners and sugars
- Shellfish
- Instant coffee
- Many gluten-free cross-contaminating foods (found in gluten-free products), such as:
    - Corn
    - Rice
    - Potato Starch
    - Tapioca

- Buckwheat
- Quinoa
- Sesame
- Oats
- Teff
- Rye
- Yeast

No, not ALL of these foods are off limits, but if your tummy is troubled, consider if any of these are a regular part of your diet. Many of these foods contain various types of proteins or components that are more difficult to digest.

The good news? The pain associated with certain trigger foods doesn't have to last forever, and more than anything, can be a good indicator that there is some "gut work" to be done (like the 28 day reset). Be a sleuth and if stomach issues are your "norm," evaluate your own daily intake and question what offenders—even healthy foods—may be driving a stress response in your gut.

3. Chronic Undereating

Much of our culture is hyperfocused on overeating. However, lack of enough fuel each day sends your body into "stressed-out" mode just as much as overeating.

Whether you lose your appetite when you're worried or mentally stressed, you're on a diet, or simply don't eat enough due to sluggish digestion, a busy schedule or "forgetting to eat," when you fail to meet your nutrient and energy needs, your body is forced to make do the best it can with what it does get. Common indicators that you may be chronically undereating:

- Difficulty losing inches, gaining muscle, or shifting body composition
- Loss of appetite or feelings of hunger

- Fatigue or low energy
- Decreased digestion
- Constipation, bloating, gas or abdominal cramping when you do eat
- Quickly full after eating
- Brain fog
- Feeling easily run down
- Thinking about food often
- Hormonal imbalances (loss of period, crazy PMS)
- Plateaus in the gym
- Adrenal insufficiency
- Headaches
- Dips and crashes during the day
- Lowered immune function
- Allergy sensitivities
- Lowered libido

The Minnesota Starvation study (Keys et al, 1950) is one of the most popular studies, and revealed what chronic undereating does to the normal human body.

In it, 36 normal weight men underwent six weeks of restricted eating, during which researchers observed a myriad of both mental and physical stresses (anxiety, lowered energy, apathy, elevated emotions, weakness) which led to chronic stress, *even* during the re-feeding process when participants were able to eat enough again (Kalm & Semba, 2005). In short: The men learned to live in the stressed-out state, and their stress hormones (cortisol) and metabolisms adapted accordingly. Likewise, undereating forces your body and gut to adapt to a state of chronic stressed.

4. Low Carb Intake

Low carb diets are extremely popular. Diet ads and low carb advocates claim that carbs make us fat and sugar is the enemy.

However, just like high sugar consumption is equally a stressor for the gut, so is lack of carbohydrate energy.

The human body needs a balance of all macro-nutrients for optimal health.

While low carb diets, low-fat diets **or** low protein (vegan/vegetarian) diets can be beneficial for some people as a nutritional or therapeutic diet (depending on their body's health state or needs), a combination of protein, fat and carbohydrates is needed overall. All three provide the body with different essentials for optimal health over the long haul.

Low carb diets, in particular, lack fiber—specifically prebiotic fiber and resistant starch. Fiber and carbs from some starchy tubers and **prebiotic** foods (cooked and cooled potatoes, green-tipped bananas and plantains) help promote healthy digestion by moving bulk in our stool from one end to the other.

Hence, lower-carb, higher-fat and/or higher protein diets can do the opposite (i.e. cause constipation). Even if you ARE eating lots of leafy greens, it may not be enough to push it all through the hose.

A common roadblock folks run into when switching to a "real food" or "quality" food diet is the trap of accidental dieting. They naturally decrease their carb intake—cutting the typical Standard American grain-based diet they once ate.

The problem? Many fail to replace these carbs with more real-food carbs—starchy tubers, fruits and veggies—or *enough* fuel from other sources (enough fat, enough protein). Easily one's intake can become eggs and bacon for breakfast, chicken and salad for lunch, and salmon and broccoli for dinner—very low carb.

Without enough fuel to add to the "fire" of energy demands, the body gets stressed.

A review of seven studies (McGrice & Porter, 2017) on the impact of low carb diets on women's hormones found that, in generally healthy women, hormones become imbalanced with low carb dieting (i.e. loss of period, suppressed estrogen and testosterone levels, infertility). The average human who is moderately active (both inside and outside the gym) needs carbohydrates, just as much as she or he needs proteins or fats—with the bulk of these being real foods that your gut knows how to digest.

5. Sugar

Sugar is everywhere. The average American consumes 3 pounds of sugar each week—a stark difference from the Americans in 1900 who consumed 10 pounds of sugar every year.

Sugar is not just found in Hershey's candy bars or other sweets, but also in salad dressings, breads, pastas, sauces, crackers, yogurts, granola bars, sports drinks, protein powders, mustards, and deli meats.

Sugar is not innately bad (the body can handle a little bit of chocolate every now and then), but high consumption of sugar and hidden sugars (even artificial sweeteners) elevates your cortisol levels (stress). Cortisol LOVES sugar (in fact, it feeds off of it for an adrenaline rush). If you experience frequent sugar cravings or blood sugar imbalances, chances are cortisol is pulling on your shirt tail.

Common signs of blood sugar imbalances include:

- Shakiness between meals or getting "hangry" if you go too long between meals
- High need to snack between meals
- Headaches
- Afternoon crashes or sleepiness
- 10 a.m.—mid-morning—cravings

- Insomnia or broken sleep
- Frequent thirst or urination
- Family members who have diabetes
- Binging or uncontrolled/emotional eating
- Coffee
- Sugar cravings

Ideally, your body was wired to be "fat burner"—not a sugar burner—able to run off fats as its main source of fuel and energy, relying less on sugar as the primary driver. Modern society has raised many of us to be the opposite.

As kids, many of us grew up eating Goldfish snack crackers, Oreos and fruit yogurts—high carb and sugar-based diets—with a palate for more "quick energy" sources (like pizza, quesadillas and PB&J's—as opposed to avocados, nuts and seeds, and well-balanced, veggie, protein and fat-based meals).

Adults aren't much different. The bulk of American diets is low in veggies (1 in 10 gets the recommended servings), low in healthy fats, moderate in proteins and high in short-burst carbohydrate fuel—even "clean diet foods" (i.e. bars, yogurts, Quest bars, cereals, whole grains, beans, crackers, muffins, fruits).

Lack of balance turns the body into "sugar burning" (and sugar craving) mode, demanding you eat more of these sugar-based foods (i.e. low fat, snacks and grain or carb-based fuel) to keep going.

In addition, gut bacteria feed off and thrive on sugar, refined carbohydrates and even some starchy veggies and fruits, like FODMAPS.

Consequently when your gut bugs are hungry, sugar cravings may strike.

Diets higher in sugar, FODMAP fruits and veggies, starches and grains can lead to GI dysfunction if you have bacterial overgrowth. Grains in particular (even whole grains gluten free grains, like rice and oats, as well as legumes) also contain components called "anti-nutrients" on their outer shell called *lectins* and *phytates*. Lectins and phytates are meant to protect plants from weather conditions, as well as predators in the wild. When our human gut consumes them consistently, it has difficulty breaking them down. These anti-nutrients also bind to other vitamins and minerals, preventing absorption of many of the nutrients in your food in the first place.

Q. So should I just cut the carbs?!

A. Not so fast. Complete carb elimination is not necessarily the answer either. In fact, gut bacteria and yeast, like Candida, can equally feast and feed on high-fat (i.e. ketogenic) diets and ketones (Beier et al, 2014), and higher-protein, lower-carb diets can equally wreak havoc on the gut, primarily because they often neglect essential prebiotic fiber and starchy tuber fibers to help push food through your digestive tract. However, some people find they do benefit from experimenting with low-FODMAP based diets while trying to get to the root of their gut issues.

FODMAP 101

FODMAP is an acronym for a collection of foods that contain certain short-chain carbohydrates and sugar alcohols which can activate gut-related symptoms due to their ability to breed and feed unhealthy gut bacteria. FODMAP stands for **fermentable, oligosaccharides, disaccharides, monosaccharides and polyols**. Basically, FODMAPS are sugars, starches, and fibers that unhealthy gut bacteria thrive on. If you experience irritable bowel syndrome, bloating or constipation, consider eliminating high FODMAP foods from your diet to see how you feel.

High FODMAP Foods

- **Vegetables:** artichoke, asparagus, broccoli, brussels sprouts, cabbage, cauliflower, garlic, leek, onion, shallot, snow peas, tomato/tomato paste
- **Fruits:** apple, apricot, cherry, mango, peach, pear, plum, watermelon, avocado (in large quantities)
- **Beans:** legumes (lentils, beans, peanuts) and soy
- **Fats:** vegetable oils and inflammatory omega-6 fats like canola, soybean and peanut oil
- **Nuts and seeds:** pistachios, almonds and hazelnuts
- **All grains and dairy products, alcohol and sugars,** including natural sugars and artificial sweeteners, are considered high FODMAP foods.

Low FODMAP Foods

- **Vegetables**: beet, bok choy, carrot, cucumber, endive, kale, lettuce, olives, spinach, Swiss chard, winter squash
- **Fruits**: banana, blueberries, kiwi, orange, pineapple, raspberries, rhubarb, strawberries, plantains
- **Proteins**: muscle and organ meats, fish, seafood, eggs, bone broth
- **Fats**: avocado oil, coconut oil, ghee, cod liver oil, olive oil

Every BODY reacts differently, and all FODMAPS may not be completely off limits. Experiment to find what works for you.

Note: If you are actively treating SIBO, fungal, parasitic or bacterial infection with an antimicrobial herbal treatment or antifungal antibiotics (like Rifaximin), a low FODMAP diet may not be necessary. FODMAP foods encourage gut bacteria to "come out" so your antimicrobial treatment can go to work.

6. Poor Food Hygiene.

Food hygiene, like self-care hygiene, involves the basic principles of "self-care" from a digestive standpoint:

- Slowing down at meals (rest and digest)
- Breathing before meals
- Chewing your food thoroughly
- Preparing and handling a vast majority of your own food at home
- Knowing where your food comes from
- Eating fresh food in season—as much as possible
- Washing your hands and foods before prepping
- Storing food in glassware containers
- Not drinking fluids with meals (may sip) for optimal digestive juices
- Mindful Eating and Vitamin P (below)
- Giving thanks for your food

The word "hygiene" itself means *"conditions or practices conducive to maintaining health and preventing disease, especially through cleanliness."*

So food hygiene is the practice of maintaining the best digestible, nutrient-dense food as possible.

It helps eliminate stress from the digestive process and enhances the quality of your food you put in your mouth, beyond foods simply labeled "healthy" or "good for you."

Remember, optimal digestion happens in the parasympathetic mode—rest and digest. If you were running from that bear in the open fields, the last thing your body is thinking about is eating food.

Even though we don't commonly run from bears these days, we sort of do when we eat on the go in our car, eat mindlessly in front of the TV, inhale our food, or fail to chew our food. Chewing your food *well* is particularly important in the context of digestion.

Chewing assists in breaking down your food from large particles into smaller particles which are more easily digested—making the whole process of digestion much smoother. Chewing also increases the amount of digestive enzymes, like lipase and amylase, that accumulate in your saliva. The longer you chew, the *more* enzyme activity you have to help break down your food—also assisting in smoother digestion.

Unfortunately, many people do three things when they eat: Chew. Chew. Swallow. (Repeat). No need to count the number of bites, but mindfully think about taking smaller bites, fully breaking down that food until you no longer recognize the food it was before, finish chewing completely before swallowing and…. breathe.

Aside from chewing, also consider *how* you eat, where you eat and your food preparation process. Do you eat in a hurry? Forget to breathe or taste and savor your food? Wash your hands before a meal? Know what oils were used in the kitchen to prep your food? Connect to your food—do you know where it was grown or cultivated?

All of these factors can play a positive role in boosting digestion naturally. How can you maximize your food hygiene? Pick one to start.

7. Vitamin P Deficiency

Did you know that if you lack pleasure from food—Vitamin P—your stress levels actually increase? No matter how "clean" you eat, if you really hate that dry salad, egg whites, or chicken breast, then so does your body—digestion included.

Studies (Yau & Potenza, 2013) have revealed the "negative" sides of pleasure from foods on health—such as the brain chemicals that light up (like a person on drugs) when you eat sugar, or the addicting effects of Doritos. However, fewer explore how a healthy relationship with foods we eat (and pleasure from those foods) can positively influence health and digestion.

A group of researchers from the University of Texas (Psychology of Eating, 2013) tackled this in a study, finding that people's metabolisms are actually **not** affected as "negatively" as believed when they ate foods they enjoyed—even if they weren't the healthiest foods.

While we've discussed the importance of food quality and real food for good digestion, that does not discount the equal importance of finding pleasure and peace with food. Fueling your body with "good fuel" does not have to be a laborious chore and quality fuel + food you enjoy (even the occasional slice of pizza) does a body (and mind) good.

It's all about balance.

In fact, one study (Scelzo, 2018) found the "secret" to living past 100 years old includes eating a rich, flavorful diet in a variety of proteins—fish, chicken and beef, vegetables (especially leafy greens), lots of healthy fats, wine, and limiting sugar, pasta and pizza to once per week (but still being able to eat it).

You CAN have your cake and eat it too, and when you do, your stress levels (and gut health), ironically, may improve.

8. Coffee

Do you…

Need coffee to function?
Need coffee to poop?

Need coffee to wake up and feel human?
Need coffee to 'keep going?'
Need coffee to 'calm down' or keep alert?
Get headaches if you don't have coffee (or caffeine)?
Get jittery if you have coffee (or don't have any)?
Experience "crashes" during the day—only relieved by coffee or sugar?
Get wired and tired at night?

If you answered 'yes' to any of these, chances are you may have trained your body (and mind) to become dependent on coffee. While coffee is not inherently a bad thing—it's when we "need" coffee that things may go a little haywire in our own skin.

The average American drinks at least two to three cups of coffee per day, and coffee (and caffeine) have a major impact on your body's stress levels (i.e. cortisol) and your HPA-Axis by and large. (No wonder we are all stressed!).

Your HPA-Axis (hypothalamic pituitary adrenal (HPA) axis) is the "mothership" of stress, otherwise known as your "**central stress response system.**"

When it is confronted with a stressor—like coffee—it reacts in order to protect you.

Drink coffee—>Elevate cortisol.

Coffee intake (even just 200 mg—the amount in a 12 oz. cup of coffee) can spike cortisol levels by 30%. Moreover, cortisol can remain elevated for up to 18 hours in the blood (meaning we already put ourselves in a deficit, if we are drinking our first cup of coffee with breakfast, followed by another cup or shot of espresso three to six hours later).

Although cortisol is a natural *necessary* stress hormone (designed to help you wake up in the morning, endure a tough workout, handle the stress of a boss's negative feedback and cope with in emergencies when in danger), when we elevate it beyond what it can handle, things go awry.

Unwanted elevated cortisol is directly associated with side effects like increased anxiety, stubborn metabolism or weight gain, disrupted sleep, poor recovery from workouts, increased fatigue, hormonal imbalances, suppressed appetite or insatiable appetite, lowered immunity and sugar cravings.

So imagine what happens if day in and day out, we continue to drink it (sometimes even several times per day)?

We continue to raise cortisol.

In addition to being a natural stressor, coffee also happens to be one of the **moldiest foods** we consume—particularly instant coffee. In fact, instant coffee is one of the most cross-contaminating foods with gluten, pointing to gut health imbalances.

9. Screen Time

Artificial light—particularly from the blue light found in computer and phone screens—has a huge influence on your stress levels. For the vast majority of humans' evolutionary history, we lived in harmony with the natural rhythms of day and night, without exposure to artificial light—cell phones and other devices included. Today, the average American spends more than 10 hours on a screen each day between cell phones, computers and TVs (Nielson Report, 2016).

Artificial light (both screens and light bulbs) has the *strongest* influence on your circadian system, and yet, an estimated 95 percent of Americans regularly use screens shortly before going to sleep. Light exposure to both screens and fake light inside has been shown to *shift* your natural human biological clock—delaying the effect and quality of sleep, as well as recovery, gut detoxification and metabolic processes that happen when we sleep—crucial for a "healthy gut." For instance, **one study** (Phipps-Nelson et al, 2003), revealed that an hour of "normal" moderately bright light exposure (1,000 lux) was sufficient to suppress nocturnal melatonin to daytime levels (i.e. keep you awake).

While it's difficult to imagine life *without* screens today, recognition of when we use them, taking breaks, getting as much outdoor exposure and natural light as possible, and using blue-light-dimming apps (Like "Nightshift" and "f.lux") are proactive measures we can take to diminish screen time.

Circadian Rhythm Disruption

Undersleeping is a modern day epidemic. One-third of all Americans get less than six hours of sleep per night—an equivalency on our brain levels as being legally intoxicated (Jang-Young et al, 2015). Without enough sleep, our body is unable to complete the full process of elimination and digestion (when waste is typically created)—and constipation, bloating and gas may be directly linked to your lack of shut eye.

Couple this with shift work—working at odd hours of the day (when the body is physiologically preparing for sleep and is required to sleep when performance, alertness, and core body temperature are on the rise) is also a stressor.

Approximately 20 percent of people in the industrialized world work beyond the "normal" day shift in various schedules of shift work. From police officers and firefighters to store managers, on-call customer service representatives, or the job of being a college student (and the all-nighters we pulled back in the day), shift work messes with circadian rhythm function, which messes with digestion and gut health.

10. Treadmills & Couches

Too much or too little of a good thing is not a good thing. With exercise, we want the "Goldilocks" approach—just right. Exercise IS a natural stressor, and the "just right" amount can yield positive health and results if you stay within an appropriate threshold.

However, if your body is *over-stressed* from either training beyond its capacity to recover or never moving at all, then you will reap the consequences—like poor ability to "keep up" with training (or see results). Like a bank account, we each only have a select amount of "stress" dollars to spend before we run dry—and then we're left spinning our wheels, in poor health, no results or falling short in our workout efforts (even though "we are doing everything right").

Each body has a unique threshold of just how much stress it can handle—and what stress looks like for each person is uniquely different, depending on what else you have going on in your life. On this note, there is no one-size-fits-all approach for finding the "just right balance" for your training.

For some, *less is more,* and for others, some can handle or need more fitness in their life. The biggest indicator of if you are over-training or not is to simply address the facts (no crazy lab work even needed on this one): Are you thriving?

Some common indicators of too much treadmill (or workout) time include:

- Continued digestive problems, despite healthy digestive practices
- Plateaus in your fitness or strength
- Slowed metabolism
- Hypermetabolism (can't "keep up" with the demands of your body)

- Stubborn body fat
- Constantly thinking about food or exercise
- Actively restricting calories or food groups
- Dreading your workouts
- Feeling compelled by your workouts
- Counting calories in your workouts
- Apathy
- Anxiety—especially if or when you don't get your workout in
- Thinking about the end of your workout—even when you've just started
- Not knowing what to do if you don't workout
- Missing social events or sleep often times for a workout
- Using caffeine or energy drinks to keep going
- Achy joints
- Injuries
- Never feeling "sore" or challenged by your workouts (spinning your wheels)
- Viewing your workouts like a checklist
- Never varying your workout types or intensity

11. Indoor Recess

Lack of sunshine and fresh air is a huge force working against the natural circadian rhythms and health balance of your body. Humans were designed to live in nature.

Although we are thankful for roofs over our head and air conditioning in the 90-100 degree temperatures of summertime, modern day evolution still does not replace our innate human need for fresh air. Couple this with 8-12 hours of time spent indoors, staring at screens (work, TV, phones and computers), and our bodies get extra stressed.

Do you remember indoor recess as a kid? It was definitely not as much fun as outdoor recess—where all the swings and kickball field, slides and soccer balls were. Indoor recess meant board games, reading, or climbing the walls.

Your body feels the same way without that extra bit of fresh air. If anything, Vitamin D from the sun is crucial for overall health, and low Vitamin D is associated with fatigue, hypothyroidism, hormone imbalances, fatigue, nutrient deficiencies and digestive dysfunction.

In addition, lack of play itself is another stressor. Our society tends to dismiss play for adults. Play is perceived as unproductive, petty or even a guilty pleasure.

Modern day humans are *really good* at "playing" on the computer, devices, watching TV and being entertained. The average American adult spends upwards of 12 hours sitting each day (JustStand.org, 2017)—much of this at screens or in traffic—detracting from time spent playing, moving, creating, exploring, experiencing and stimulating our brains (in other ways outside data spreadsheets and social media posts).

Get this: Lack of play was just as important as other factors in predicting criminal behavior among murderers in Texas prisons. Play also helps build relationships—studies of couples who play together shows play helps to rekindle their relationship and explore other forms of emotional intimacy (Brown, 2010). And in older adults, those who incorporate play and pleasurable daily activities into their physical activity are more likely to stick with exercise than those who do not—leading to better health outcomes.

And, if you want the best of both worlds, couple play with outdoor play and you have a double whammy. A study in the *International Journal of Environmental Research and Public Health*,

(Brussoni, 2015) found that children who participated in "risky" physical activity such as climbing and jumping, rough and tumble play, and exploring alone, displayed greater physical and social health. The study author noted that play environments where children could take risks promoted increased play time, social interactions, creativity and resilience.

Similar to kids, when adults incorporate play (i.e. social connection, entertainment, game play, creative play, fitness, adventures, hobbies and respite activities), it relieves stress, boosts creativity, improves brain function, and improves relationships with other people by fostering trust with others.

12. Facebook, Instagram & Snapchat

The rapid development of social networking sites such as Facebook, Instagram, Snapchat, and others has caused several profound changes in the way people communicate, interact and how they feel about themselves. With more than one billion people on Facebook alone, we are constantly bombarded with updates and pressures to get more likes, notifications, and to see—and be seen—by others on the interwebs.

A survey conducted by Glamour Magazine (Dreisbach, 2014) found that 64 percent of women walk away from social media feeling worse about themselves—not better—after comparing themselves to others. Another study of nearly 24,000 people found the same thing, citing addictive social media use to be common amongst people, and serves as both a consequence and a predictor of low self-esteem (Andreassen et al, 2017).

Some people also use social media to feel better about themselves. For example, if an individual thinks "I am not likable" or "I have poor social skills" – while at the same time believing that having a large number of friends or followers will change such self-evaluations, than he or she is more likely to turn to the screen to find validation.

The problem is, *we will never have enough friends, likes or followers*—social media is a continual dangling carrot and can serve as a driving force of stress in our lives unbeknownst to us until we check in with ourselves.

The average American is on their phone within the first five minutes of waking (Deloitte, 2016), checking their social media newsfeed and emails. Before you've had time to say your prayers or morning meditations! Get your mind right with positivity or get some energy flowing with movement, BEFORE your brain is influxed with the comparisons and stresses of "measuring up" (or down) on social media.

13. Disconnection

Hand in hand with our lack of face-to-face time with others, due to the viral growth and usage of social media, disconnection with people and community is another source of stress which can wreak havoc on your overall well-being.

Social connections are like green juice, bone broth, and probiotics - it's an important element in overall health.

People without strong social ties are more at risk for a host of inflammatory conditions, including the development and progression of cardiovascular disease, recurrent myocardial infarction, atherosclerosis, autonomic dysregulation, high blood pressure, cancer and delayed cancer recovery, and slower wound healing (Ertel et al, 2009; Everson-Rose & Lewis 2005; Robles and Kiecolt-Glaser 2003; Uchino 2006). In addition, a survey showed that lack of social connectedness predicts vulnerability to disease and death above and beyond traditional risk factors such as smoking, blood pressure, and physical activity.

Thinking back to our ancestors, who lived in communities and had close knit relationships with others, we are living in a society where now, more than ever, we are disconnected.

Research on the subject of human disconnection has found that while we are seemingly more connected nowadays thanks to social media and constant communication on our phones and online platforms, people are less engaged when physically together. More than 75 percent of women and 50 percent of men check their phones and social media news feeds more than 10 times when together in a social environment, and nearly 90 percent admit to missing out on conversation simply due to distraction by their phones (Saiidi, 2015).

One of the most popular studies (Egolf et al, 1992) on the power of human connection and relationships involves the community of Roseto, Pennsylvania.

In this small town, researchers noted that the Roseto people were some of the "unhealthiest" people around—they smoked, they drank, worked long hours, and ate lots of processed meats—and yet, researchers could not understand why Roseto people lived longer and did not contract heart disease like many of the communities around them.

The Roseto people had one of the lowest rates of deaths by heart attacks—practically none—during the 10-year research period, and the only outlier the researchers could conclude was that the Roseto people lived in—and highly valued—community connections. Rosetans lived with their families and loved ones in tight-knit circles and spent many of their non-working hours cultivating relationships, play, and experiences with other people.

Research on the "blue zones"—the healthiest cities in the world—also show similar findings. Generally in the cities where people report living the longest and being happier and healthier overall, they are living in communities where connection to other humans and interaction with their environment are integral parts of daily culture. In other words, social media in a blue zone means getting together and talking with friends or drinking tea together.

Beyond just waking up, going to work, then coming home to make dinner and watch TV, the blue zones are generally walkable communities where active lifestyles are a given, communities are bustling and people get out with other people.

Conversely, negative relationships equally impact our stress levels—in a negative way (Kagamimori et al, 2004). Whether it's an abusive relationship, a job environment you dislike, or the burden of caring for an aging loved one, relationships can also be a source of stress if we don't actively seek to counter that stress with positive influences in our lives. There's a saying which goes, "You are the sum of the five people you surround yourself with. Make 'em good."

Don't neglect the role community can play in your own stress suppression and gut health (believe it or not).

14. Environmental Toxins

We live in a toxic world. According to the Environmental Working Group (Benesh, 2016) more than 85,000 fake chemicals, additives and toxins have been "approved" by the U.S. Environmental Protection Agency to be used in our foods, cleaning products, beauty products and environmental surroundings, with about 2,000 more being added *every year.*

And, while they say we are "safe" around these chemicals and toxins, more and more research continues to point to the opposite.

When we are exposed to harsh chemicals and toxins, we run the risk of disrupting our endocrine and hormone balance, undermining our thyroid health, challenging our immunity, and, yes, throwing off our digestion. Similar to the "wear and tear" on our digestive tract we've talked about, toxic exposure is not always *seen* with the naked human eye, but equally does a number on the integrity of our gut and risk for bacterial overgrowth.

Review this questionnaire and see where you fall on the spectrum of being affected by toxic exposure and the world around you. Answer 'yes' or 'no' to each question.

- Do you consume conventionally grown (non-organic) fruits and vegetables, farmed seafood or conventional animal meats regularly?
- Do you consume fast foods, canned/packaged foods, soda, or foods with artificial colors, flavors, preservatives or sweeteners more than three times a week?
- Have you lived in a very old or brand-new apartment/home?
- Have you recently been exposed to new construction materials or furniture (e.g., paint, laminate
- flooring, particle board, new carpeting, bedding, furniture, etc.)?
- Is there a presence of musty smells in your environment?
- Have you ever traveled out of the country and become sick?
- Does your home or workplace have cracking paint or decaying insulation or foam, visible mold, water damage, or damp windows, basement, or crawl spaces?
- Are you often exposed to adhesives, paints, flea treatments, varnishes, solvents, welding/soldering materials, or other airborne chemicals at home or work?
- Do you regularly use conventional cleaning chemicals, disinfectants, hand sanitizers, air fresheners, scented candles, or other scented products at home or work?

- Are you highly sensitive to smoke, perfumes, fragrances, cleaning products, gasoline, or other fumes?
- Have you had root canals, tooth extractions, "silver" fillings, crowns, dental sealants, dentures, retainers, aligning trays, braces, mouthguards, dental implants, etc.?
- Do you have a history of heavy use of alcohol, recreational drugs, or prescription drugs?
- Do you smoke or are you regularly exposed to secondhand smoke?
- Do you use plastic tupperware or drink from plastic water bottles regularly?
- Do you drink tap water?
- Have you had any unusual reactions to anesthesia or to prescription or over-the-counter medications?
- Do you live near a cell phone tower, high-voltage power lines, or other known source of electromagnetic radiation?
- Have you taken antibiotics at some point in your life for more than one month?
- Do you regularly consume NSAIDs?
- Have you taken a prescription medication for longer than three months?

If you answered 'yes' to more than five of these, you're more at risk for toxic exposure stress on your gut. For instance, antibiotics in our conventional food sources or medications have the ability to eradicate (destroy) colonies of good bacteria: they wipe out the good guys along with the bad.

"Toxic exposure" does not have to involve traveling to a third-world country, either, or a bad case of food poisoning. It can stem from the simplest of things that we use or consume every day:

- Beauty products we use every morning (our skin eats what we put on it!)

- Additives in your Diet Coke or artificially-sweetened protein powders and bars
- Shellac nail polish at the salon
- The salmon you cooked last night or the tuna fish you ate at lunch
- Alcohol in our skin toner
- An overcooked burger at the 4th of July cookout
- Sunscreens
- Secondhand smoke
- The water you drank from the water fountain at the YMCA
- The hand-sanitizer you keep in your purse
- The toothpaste you've used since you were a kid
- GMOs in our fruits and veggies
- Antibiotics and hormones in our conventional meats at the restaurant
- Plastic water bottles and Tupperware

In fact, according to an assessment by the Environmental Working Group's Skin Deep Initiative, of more than 2,000 products we use daily (hygiene and cleaning), more than half did NOT adequately disclose ingredients, 75 percent contained ingredients that have "worrisome health effects," and 25 percent scored moderate to high concern, with ingredients in the products which have been linked to cancer.

Another **study** (Kwa et al, 2017) published in the *JAMA Journal of Internal Medicine* analyzed reports received by the Food and Drug Administration concerning "adverse events and bad reactions" to cosmetics between 2004 and 2016, finding that 5,144 adverse events were reported during that time frame, (with baby products having higher than average reports). The authors also noted that, since the 5,144 reviewed reports were entirely voluntary, they are only a small picture of what the real risks are of many products we use to public health, especially in regard to children's health.

And, lastly, a survey by the Centers for Disease Control and Prevention (CDC, 2010) found traces of 212 environmental chemicals in Americans themselves — including toxic metals like arsenic and cadmium, pesticides, flame retardants and perchlorate (an ingredient in rocket fuel).

15. Antibiotics

Antibiotics are regarded as miracle drugs by many, however, they actually may be making you more sick in the long run. Here's what you need to know about antibiotics and how they impact your gut and overall health.

Chances are, if you're an American, you've taken an antibiotic at one time or another. We are overly exposed to antibiotics throughout our lifetimes, due not only to medical use, but also to antibiotic utilization in farm animals and crops. Prescribed by most doctors to cure "everything"—from a cold to an ear infection, acne, strep throat, food poisoning, allergy attack and everything in between—antibiotics are often viewed as the first line of defense for "feeling better." In fact, more than 40 percent of all people believe antibiotics are the best way to treat illness—especially fevers, sore throats, and runny noses (Carter et al, 2016).

No wonder four out of five people take an antibiotic every year (CDC, 2017)--even though one in three antibiotic prescriptions are actually deemed "useless" (as in: *not necessary* for the disease) according to studies (CDC, 2016)!

So what's the big deal with antibiotics?

Antibiotics may be doing more harm than good.

Three words: Destroy gut bacteria.

Antibiotics, also known as antibacterials, are medications which destroy or slow down the growth of bacteria, such as a specific flu virus or salmonella in your GI Tract. When you take an antibiotic, it enters your bloodstream and travels through your body killing bacteria, but not human cells.

However, while it may seem like a GOOD thing to destroy the bacteria associated with your current sore throat, antibiotics take NO prisoners. Antibiotic drugs don't just kill off the pathogenic ("bad") bacteria associated with the one illness you're battling, but they ALSO kill off or disrupt healthy, thriving bacteria—especially in your gut.

Microbiome composition can be rapidly altered by exposure to antibiotics, with potential immediate effects on health, for instance, through killing off bacteria and cells which otherwise typically prevent pathogens from causing acute diseases—like a lingering cold that won't go away, or sudden flare of allergies you never had before.Other side effects are not as immediate.

Over time, antibiotics can also cause a phenomenon known as "antibiotic resistance"—when antibiotics NO LONGER work as intended.

If you've ever taken a round of antibiotics to "cure" a disease, then repeated the same treatment for your cold the following year and discovered the antibiotic did NOT work like it did the first time, you're not crazy. Sort of like the idea behind a flu shot (i.e. you get the shot, and become "superhuman" to catching the flu), antibiotic resistance happens when bacteria become resistant to every type of treatment after repeat exposure to antibiotics (i.e. they can't be killed).

The result?

Not only is your immune system weakened, but pathogenic ("bad") gut bacteria can begin to take over the "good guys," setting the stage for a host of potential (longer term) side effects, including:

- SIBO (small intestinal bacterial overgrowth)
- Leaky gut
- Fungal and/or bacterial infection
- Other gut-related symptoms (hormone imbalances, poor immune function, acne, low energy, high cholesterol and inflammation, slowed metabolism, brain fog, anxiety)

Beyond antibiotics, other studies reveal that approximately one in three other medications--including antibacterials, statins, PPIs and SSRIs also disrupt the gut microbiome (Maier et al, 2018).

16. Rainy ("Bad") Days

"Hard days" are bound to come, and traumas—such as the death of a loved one, surgeries, car accidents, sports injuries or a horrible breakup—are all sources of stress which can be an extra trigger to push our bodies and gut health over the edge.

You could be getting along just fine—despite under sleeping, late night screen time, occasional hydrogenated oil and sugar consumption, or a long-term smoking habit, then suffer from a debilitating back or hip injury, demanding you have surgery and be placed on a stint of antibiotics that are the "straw" that break the camel's back.

With "poor gut" health or a sudden flare of a disease, there is typically a triggering event that sets the body off, and sometimes a trauma is at play.

17. Burning a Candle at Both Ends

"There's never enough time in the day," #SaidMostPeople.

"Hurry Syndrome" is a common phenomenon in a world where instant gratification is for real. Instant coffee, instant photography, instant dating apps, instant movies and books, instant delivery—we are constantly on the go.

Is your Hurry Syndrome a source of your gut stress?

This is often where mental stress comes into play.

Remember, 90 percent of serotonin (your feel-good brain chemical which regulates anxiety, happiness, and mood) is produced in your gut alone. So, when you get hyped up and stressed out about "getting more done," or fear "missing out" (FOMO), or bite off more than you can chew in your schedule, guess what happens to that gut of yours?

It gets overtaxed and runs low on that serotonin.

In addition to "Hurry Syndrome," some other common sources of mental-driven stress include "**Yes Syndrome**" (people pleasing and saying "yes" to everyone and everything), "**Approval Syndrome**" (looking to others for validation, likes on social media, or inclusion), "**Perfectionist Syndrome**" (needing to be perfect), and straight up classic **anxiety**.

18. The Brain-Gut Connection

This is the brain-gut connection - when the anxiety or stress you feel in your head is directly connected (and influenced) by your gut.

The mind and body are **not** separate.

The stress you feel *upstairs (in your head)* impacts the stress you feel *downstairs (in your gut)*.

Often referred to as the "second brain," it is the only organ that boasts its own independent nervous system—a network of 100 million neurons embedded in the gut wall.

Your gut bacteria are responsible for producing the hundreds of neurochemicals your brain uses to regulate basic physiological processes and mental processes such as learning, memory, mood, and anxiety management. In fact, research (Berick, 2011) has found, for example, that tweaking the balance between beneficial and disease-causing bacteria in an animal's gut can alter its brain chemistry and lead it to become either more bold or more anxious.

In addition, given the brain is the key organ of stress processes, your mindset can ALSO greatly influence your gut health.

Your brain determines what experiences are actually stressful or not, and it orchestrates how you cope with stressful experiences—changing your body chemistry (and gut function) as a result of stressful experiences.

Low self-esteem, negative thinking, worry, anxiety, and mental stress worsen digestive distress and vice versa (positive thinking improves digestive stress!).

Ever had butterflies in your stomach—the feeling of your mental nerves, physically?

We've talked a lot about external and physical stressors—like the foods you eat and toxins you are around—but mental stress should not be discounted.

Call it "Type A" personalities, people-pleasers, go-getters or procrastinators. When you stress out mentally, your body feels it. For example, at least one-third of people with anxiety and depression experience bloating regularly (Hosseinzadeh et al, 2011), and researchers have found a significantly strong correlation between all psychiatric categories (ADD and ADHD, eating disorders, anxiety, depression, etc.) and chronic constipation

Conversely, other studies have seen the *positive impacts* that **positivity** and **mindfulness** can play in you health—gut health included. One study (Vlieger et al, 2012) of 49 patients with IBS found that hypnotherapy treatment (changing their mindset)

was more beneficial than "standard" medical protocols for influencing gut health, with two-thirds of patients still in remission from symptoms five years later. The same results were also reported in those with depression (Dwivedi & Kotnala, 2014). Cognitive Behavioral Therapy (CBT) and Mindfulness Based Therapy (Ballou & Keefer, 2017) are two other leading treatments for IBS patients—superior to basic support and medical treatments for improving bowel symptoms, quality of life, and psychological stress. (Jessurun et al, 2016).

The bottom line?
How you think *does* influence your gut health, and vice versa.

While the physical stressors we've discussed are often overlooked factors in the state of your gut health, do not discount the power of your mindset in your own gut love project (this is gonna be good).

19. Unintuitive/Not Going with Your Gut

You were born with the innate ability to "go with your gut." Intuition.

We often hear the word "intuition" and think "intuitive eating"—which is part of it, but not the whole story.

Intuition means "the ability to understand something immediately, without the need for conscious reasoning." The ability to know what it is you love and what you are meant to do—no questions asked. Whether you call it a "gut feeling," an "inner voice" or a "sixth sense," intuition can play a real part in our daily lifestyle choices and all around health—especially the way we spend our time.

Unfortunately, today, just like we've become disconnected with other things (like our bodies, nature, play and other people), we are also disconnected from our ability to listen to our gut and follow our heart.

- We create bucket lists with "dream" checkboxes of things we want to do—like travel, write a book, or learn to play guitar.
- We know we don't feel great when we eat eggs, or we wonder if our low energy is related to under-eating—but we keep eating the same things most days.
- We think about taking up yoga or photography, but resort to channel surfing and overworking instead.
- Our 5 a.m. alarm goes off like it does everyday, and without question, we're out the door for our usual six-mile run or HIIT workout—even if we slept only four hours or haven't taken a day off 10 days in a row.
- We say "tomorrow" we'll make a change, or "when we feel more stable then we'll look at other career paths," but…we often stay stuck right where we are.
- We want others to like us or think highly of us and bend over backwards trying to make others happy—often at our own expense.

Habits, excuses, fears, people-pleasing, and disconnection dominates our decisions—taking the magic and spontaneity of our ancestors out of our life-arcs, and reducing our deepest passions and innate longing to "go with our gut."

Exhibit A: Hating our jobs.

A total of 85 percent of people dislike going to work (Clifton, 2017), yet they spend a majority of their days working (47 hours each week according to the Bureau of Labor Statistics in 2017), so that one day they'll be able to "someday" do something they love, retire and play golf, or check items off their bucket list. What do we do when we're not working? Of the four hours devoted to activities outside work and activities of daily living (like cooking, eating, hygiene, commuting and laundry), most Americans devote at least two to three hours of those to leisure screen time (TV and computer)—defined as the number one hobby of most adults. What about sports, creative arts, dance, outdoor play and socialization with others? A mere 30-60 minutes at most. Without time for leisure and play, we miss the benefits of having passions. A study (Pressman et al, 2009) of 1,400 people found that people who said they pursued passions and hobbies they enjoyed were healthier for all markers.

"Going with your gut" goes beyond doing activities you love. It also means things like:

- The ability to say "no" when you don't have time to take on an obligation
- Being honest with your boyfriend that "it's just not working"
- Deciding where to go to college, or whether or not to leave the job draining you
- Doing the "right thing" your gut is telling you
- Connection to that Something or Someone Greater than yourself
- Speaking your mind or speaking "truth in love" to a friend who's struggling
- Circling "C" instead of "A" on your SAT assessment—that first knee jerk reaction

Anything that involves less thinking and more connection to your gut feelings

Should Monsters

I've spent the better part of my life as a people-pleaser, do-gooder, achiever, and over-thinker. But when we try to please others, lead with our heads, or let our "should monsters" take control (more than our hearts or gut feelings), we are usually out of sync with our own wants and needs. It's not that it's bad to use your head, it's that we neglect the balance of all three components of us—mind, body, and soul.

Tons of research (McGonigal, 2011) suggests that our ability to repeatedly exert self-control (over our gut intuition) is actually quite limited. Like a muscle which tires and can no longer perform at its peak strength after a workout, our self-control is diminished by previous efforts at control, even if those efforts take place in a totally different realm.

"Not going with your gut" will poop you out.

Listening to your gut, on the other hand, makes you more confident and can actually propel you to feeling better overall.

Going with Your Gut: The Research
In an experiment of college students (Lufiyanto et al, 2016), participants were shown images of a cloud of many moving dots, which looked like the noisy "snow" you might see on an old TV. Participants had to report which general direction the cloud of dots was moving in, left or right

While subjects made these decisions, researchers presented one of their eyes with emotional photographs (positive images like puppies and negative images like snakes). through a technique called "continuous flash suppression," making the emotional photographs invisible or unconscious. In short, while the subjects made their sensory decisions, they never knew they were being presented with the emotional photographs.

In all four different experiments, researchers found that people were **able to make faster and more accurate decisions when they unconsciously viewed the emotional images.** Essentially, people's brains were able to process and utilize information from the images to intuitively "go with their gut feelings" and improve their decisions. Moreover, participants got faster as the study went on, suggesting practice makes it BETTER.

Other research shows that we become more stressed when we don't go with our gut and over time, we eventually just can't do it. We cave and fall apart inside (hello stress!). A study (Kelly et al, 2012) on people given permission to go with their gut (i.e. do the right thing), found that people who are given instructions for how to lie less in their day-to-day lives are actually *able* to lie less, and when they do, their physical health improves

Listen to and go with your gut. It usually steers you in the right direction when you turn off your over-analytical brain.

20. Lack of Gut Love

Last but not least, the "mack daddy" of all gut woes: Lack of gut love. (AKA: your "inner critic").

You (and I) are often the hardest on ourselves, and guess what? Your gut feels it.

Energy attracts energy—both negative and positive—and when you hate on your body, your gut, and yourself, your body seemingly retaliates back.

Good Enough
For as long as I can remember, I wanted to be "good enough" (at least my inner critic wanted it).

Pretty enough. Thin enough. Smart enough. Capable enough. Strong enough. Successful enough. Acceptable enough. Perfect enough.

Enough, enough, enough.

Although my inner critic's definition of "enough" slightly changed over time (for example: in 3rd grade, "enough" meant making straight A's on my multiplication tests; in 7th grade "enough" meant attention from my crush; my senior year of high school, "enough" meant getting in to my dream college, and as a twenty-something, "enough" meant landing my dream job and gaining tons of followers on Instagram), the essence of what being "enough" was really all about remained the same:

Sufficient. Plenty. No longer striving.

In my mind, if I could just be "good enough," then I'd be okay with myself.

REALITY CHECK

The reality? My inner critic's continual desire to be good "enough"—in all areas— was never fully satisfied. There was always something MORE (and better) I could do, be, look like, or achieve. There was always someone prettier than me. Smarter than me. Toner than me. More fitr than me. There was always more I could do at work. More praise to earn from my boss. More to-dos to fill my list.

Like dangling a carrot over a horse's nose to keep him moving, my inner critic's "carrots" of complete acceptance, beauty, success, fulfillment and happiness continued to dangle. Sure, I passed the math test, flirted back and forth with the boy, got into college, and landed a job (maybe not *the* one dream job), but, something deep within me was never truly at peace with myself. Consequently, my own history of gut issues and health issues went hand-in-hand with my heart-gut connection.

Until I stopped looking everywhere else to define my own standards, check boxes, and ideals of what "good enough" meant, and instead genuinely started looking inside myself, and asking myself this one question:

"What does "good enough" Lauryn really mean?"

The answer? Two things:
1. Giving myself PERMISSION to not be perfect.
2. Being 100 percent, hands down the best kickass version of myself I can. No one else. Honing my own strengths, best efforts, unique gifts, talents and dreams no one else has.

In fact, according to StrengthsFinder 2.0—a personality and strengths test people take to learn more about "who" they are—the chance that another person has the same top five themes in the same order as you is **1 in 33.4 million**. That's nearly every person in the Greater Tokyo Area -- the world's most populous metropolitan area.

That's a lot of variation!

I'm Not the Only One
Of the hundreds of women and men I've consulted with over the years on digestive health, a common theme amongst those who have "done everything right" and still cannot get to the root of their gut problems is this: unrest within themselves.

Lack of "gut love" looks different for different people, but the root of it is based on ultimately how we feel and what we think about ourselves.

Multiple studies (Juth et al, 2008; Konturek et al, 2011) have shown the negative impacts of low-self esteem on gastrointestinal disorders like inflammatory bowel disease (IBD), irritable bowel syndrome (IBS), food intolerances, stomach ulcers, and reflux (GERD).

One of the most interesting cases (Emmanuel et al, 2001) assessed 34 women between the ages of 19 and 45 who had suffered from constipation for five years or more and compared these women with those of the same age range who had no history of constipation. They asked all the "poopers" and "non-poopers" to complete self-esteem assessments.

When looking at the results, what was clearly revealed was the constipated women had a worse score for overall health and felt less assured about themselves and less confident about who they were. The constipated women also found it much harder to have close relationships with others than the non-constipated women.

Researchers also looked at rectal blood flow (the function of nerve pathways from the brain to the gut which are often affected by stress). Reduced rectal blood flow was strongly associated with anxiety, depression, bodily symptoms, and impaired social skills, as well as feeling low self-esteem The lower the self-esteem score, the lower the rectal blood flow. The researchers concluded that a woman's individual psychological makeup alters the function of the involuntary nerves which link the brain to the gut. Reduced activity of these nerves slows down gut function, resulting in constipation.

Lastly, one of the best studies on the power of the mindset to date—particularly in gut healing—happened with individuals who were experiencing severe IBS—big time gut problems (Whorwell et al, 1984).

Researchers found that long term healing was "won" when hypnotherapy—not supplements—were administered. Even more, the other controls in the study did the usual psychotherapy and took placebo pills to "heal" their gut—and did not improve at all.

What this study showed is the **power of the mindset** in our own healing and health processes is MORE than just awareness or talking about our problems—it involves warping and changing our thoughts, like hypnosis does.

That brain (and gut love) of yours is a powerful force. However, just like negative self-esteem (lack of gut love) can perpetuate our gut issues, when we boost self-esteem, health improves.

A review (Enck et al, 2012) of more than 60 studies evaluating the "power of placebo" (i.e. positive thinking) in individuals with various gut disorders and symptoms found that mindset has the power to significantly influence the symptoms we feel or don't feel. For instance, in patients with IBS and abdominal pain, *consistency and belief in their own healing and well-being* produced outcomes of more than 50 percent of patients healing, no drugs or other conventional treatments required (Pitz et al, 2005).

Another meta-analysis (Sirois et al, 2015) published in the journal *Health Psychology,* found that kindness and self-compassion—accepting yourself without judgment—is linked to better health behaviors. This analysis evaluated 15 studies of more than 3,000 people of all ages and discovered a link between self-compassion and four key health-promoting behaviors: eating better, exercising more, getting more restful sleep, and stressing less. People who were more self-compassionate practiced these health habits more often. Many of us fall into the trap of cutting ourselves down (without thinking twice about it), but the research confirms that when we do so, our health suffers.

- How does your belief (in yourself) and the way you think, speak and treat yourself impact how you feel physically?
- How does your own kindness and self-care (or lack thereof) influence the peace or unrest you feel with your health and body?

- How do you think your body "feels" that (negative or positive) energy you exude?

Reflect on what messages or negative self-talk you've been telling yourself (for far too long) which may have become your "norm."

Newsflash: Your thoughts—especially those negative thoughts—are not always true. Until we can shift our own "gut love"—from the inside out—full healing will always be around the corner. Easier said than done? Nah…

Believing You Are Good Enough
I am an original. You are an original.

Originals are worth far more than replicas or imitations of those pictures.

The Sistine Chapel mural in Vatican City in Europe is 100 percent way cooler in person in the actual chapel than in a textbook or History Channel documentary.

The same thing goes for you! You have a unique set of skills, talents, strengths, passions, dreams, and experiences which shape YOU (no one else).

Perhaps Albert Einstein said it best:

"Everybody is a genius. But if you judge a fish by its ability to climb a tree, it will live its whole life believing that it is stupid."

Are you trying to be (or believing you "should be") a bear when you are really a fish?

If there's one thing I've learned about my own body, body image and gut healing, it is: **The more I HATE on my body, the more my body FEELS IT negatively.**

When I am at unrest or picking on myself or my body like a mean bully, I tend to worry more about food, my gut health, others' opinions, or checklists of achievements (plans to follow, the perfect workouts to complete, etc.).

Whereas the more I LOVE my body—speaking words of affirmation, kindness and acceptance over it, doing things I love and that make me feel good (yoga, walks, hot showers, weights, CrossFit—but not compulsion), and nourishing my body with real whole foods (rather than calculating the foods I should put in, trying different food rule philosophies)…the MORE at peace I feel with my body—just as it is. And, ironically, the more my body seems to love me back (less digestive distress, more joy with food and variety, less fatigue or stress).

"Being enough" is truly a posture of PEACE—first and foremost with yourself.

When you lean into that wind, you are unstoppable!

Stress & Gut Love Assessment

How is stress or your self-concept impacting you and your overall gut health?

Answer the following with a rating: "How often do I…"

Never	0
Rarely	1
Sometimes	2
Often/Regularly	3
Always	4

Physical Wellbeing

Eat a whole foods-based diet rich in colorful fruits and vegetables?
Eat leafy greens every day?
Drink half my bodyweight in ounces of water?
Exercise at least 3-5 days per week for 30-60 minutes?
Take 1-2 rest days off from training?
Sleep at least 7 hours per night?
Eat less than 2-3 sweets per week?
Eat 3 balanced meals per day?
Feel nourished, healthy and strong?
Get fresh air and sunshine 30-60 minutes per day?
Watch less than 60 minutes of TV most days?
Spend less than 10-30 minutes on social media most days?
Work at my job 8 hours or less per day?
Leave work at work?
Give in to sugar cravings?
Drink 1 cup of coffee or less per day?

Have a bowel movement once per day (without needing laxatives, coffee or other outside influences)?
Listen to my body if I am tired?
Get more energy when I work out?
Never force myself to go to the gym if you truly need a rest day?
Use "recovery" modalities between workouts? (Ice baths, stretching, sauna, yoga)?
Take a probiotic?
Eat fermented foods?
Use natural/organic beauty products?
Use natural/organic cleaning supplies?
Refrain from using the microwave?
Eat fat with every meal?
Eat 1-2 starchy carbs per day?
Limit fruits to 1-2 servings per day?
Refrain from medication or NSAID use?

Emotional & Mental Well-Being
Make time to participate in things I enjoy?
Feel gratitude daily?
Have hope that things will get better?
Make my goals and dreams a priority?
Have clarity or awareness of my purpose?
Treat myself with kindness?
Read and learn from other inspiration or motivational leaders?
Share openly with a trusted friend, counselor or mentor the things on my mind?
Pray or meditate?
Journal or reflect on my thoughts and feelings?
Express myself creatively?
Talk back to my inner critic?
Feel present and able to be in the moment?
Read or listen to an inspirational book or podcast?
Do things I love?

Community/Social
Feel supported in my life?
Participate in group activities with people who share a common interest?
Spend time with people who make me laugh?
Have the ability to say "no" comfortably?
Have a close relationship with my family?
Have a dependable person who listens to me?
Do something fun with others at least once per week?
Feel like my personal life brings balance to my social life?
Can ask for help when I need it?
Can be alone without getting FOMO (fear of missing out)?
Spend time with people who make me laugh?
Can think of 5 people who are good friends or encouragers in my life?

Gut Love
I'm accepting about my own flaws and inadequacies.
When I'm feeling down, I try not to obsess or focus on everything that's wrong.
When things are going badly for me, I see the difficulties as part of life everyone goes through.
I try to be loving towards myself when I'm feeling emotional pain.
When I fail at something important to me, I try to keep things in perspective.
When I am down and out, I remind myself that there are lots of other people in the world feeling like I am.
When something upsets me, I'm in control of my feelings.
When I feel inadequate in some way, I try to remind myself that feelings of inadequacy are shared by most people.
I try to see my failings as part of the human condition.
I'm tolerant of my own flaws and inadequacies.

When I see aspects of myself I don't like, I counter my inner critic's tendency to get down on myself.
When something painful happens, I try to take a balanced view of the situation.
When I'm going through a very hard time, I give myself the caring and tenderness I need.
I try to be understanding and patient towards those aspects of my personality I don't like.
I'm beautiful.
I'm smart.
I'm worth it.

The higher your score, the better you may be at taking time for self-care, stress management and wellness in each aspect of your life. Improving your scores through the Gut Kickstart can help create more balance in your life. Stick with me.

Gut Check-In Point

1. Did this assessment bring to mind any stressors present in your life? Reflect on the stressors in your life that may have played a role in the past or present in your own gut health.

From a long-term stint of antibiotics to artificial sweetener consumption, high screen time, poor quality sleep, work-life imbalance, people pleasing, being on the go 24/7, hating on your thighs and beyond.

List out as many stressors that come to mind.

2. While you're at it, consider items on which you scored 0 or 1. How can you modify your behavior to improve your self-care practices? What goals might you need to set in order to make these changes?

CHAPTER 7

The 28 Day Gut Kickstart

Now that we've established that stress is the main culprit of all gut issues and pathologies, how can you start to feel better? (After all, we can't live in a bubble and stress will always be a part of life!)

Enter: the 28 Day Gut Kickstart, a 28-day nutrition, mindset & gut healing protocol, jam-packed with step-by-step guidance and gut-healing protocols for taking your health into your own hands.

The Gut Kickstart is divided into three different phases, including:

Phase 1: Assessment & Prep Week. Seven full days to complete your Initial Gut Kickstart Assessments and get prepped for the next 28 days of gut healing (including grocery shopping and meal prep). In addition, if you want to take things to the next level, you'll have the option to complete a "jumpstart" cleanse during the 24 to 48 hours before Day 1 starts, as well as the option to perform any additional clinical lab testing, such as a stool test, SIBO breath test, and/or blood work. (More on this later).

Phase 2: 28-Day Gut Kickstart. Let the games begin! For 28 days you will eat feel-good, anti-inflammatory foods, PLUS integrate your 5 Daily Gut Love Habits into your daily routine. You'll also have full access to "Cheat Sheet" Protocols (Resources) in case you need some extra "gut love" (i.e. supplement support).

Phase 3: Next Steps: Experiment & Maintenance. At the end of your 28-days, it's time to experiment! Phase 3 consists of re-introduction of any foods you may have missed (one at a time) and customizing a way of eating which is sustainable and works for your body. You also may want to do further gut testing at this point if your gut still needs healing. This phase is ongoing, as the goal is to eat as "least restrictive" as possible, eating a variety of nutrient-dense, real foods, while continuing your gut healing journey.

Where to begin?!

Simply implement the "action" steps associated with each phase (described below) and take each day one day at a time.

The 28 Day Gut Kickstart:
HOW IT WORKS

Phase 1: Assessments & Prep Week

In order to know where you're going, you have to know where you're coming from.

Before you embark on any dietary and lifestyle changes during your 28 Day Gut Kickstart, you will get an entire 7 days ("Prep Week") to "get prepped" for the next 28 days ahead. (Note: If you need an additional week, that is fine too!).

During Prep Week, you will:

1. **Complete Your Gut Kickstart Assessments**. Conduct your Gut Kickstart Basic Assessment to assess your current gut health. (We will re-test this at the end). You can find these beginning on Page 152.

2. **Keep a 3-day Food & Poo Log (of what you are *currently* eating)** No need to change anything drastic this week. You are going to get in touch with how you feel TODAY to have a baseline of where you started (before you feel amazing at the end of your 28-Day Reset). In this log, simply write down what you ate and any symptoms you notice before and after meals (super hungry, headaches, low energy, bloating, skin breakouts, etc.), as well as when you go (#2), and what it looks like. Do this for three days, and we will reassess at the end of your kickstart.

3. **Get Prepped.** Failing to prepare is preparing to fail. Use the first seven Prep days to:

- Grocery shop for necessary foods (See your Gut Kickstart Food List & Meal Ideas in the Index)
- Experiment and meal prep any foods you'd like to have on hand
- Wean yourself off of your "old" habits (ie. multiple cups of coffee, eating on the go not sleeping enough, etc.)
- Purchase any quality supplements to support your plan, including:

Baseline Supplement Recommendations
  - Apple Cider Vinegar or HCL Capsules (600-700 mg HCL/pepsin; Note: HCL tablets are not recommended if pregnant or taking PPI's, steroids or NSAID's like Advil regularly, use apple cider vinegar instead)
  - Herbal Tea of choice
  - Soil Based Probiotic
  - Prebiotic Fiber (partially hydrolyzed guar gum)
  - Digestive Enzymes (optional)

Optional: 24-48-Hour "Cleanse."
24-48 hours before the official Day 1 begins, you will have the option to press the "refresh" button with a modified cleanse and jumpstart your body (and gut) into your 28-Day Reset!

This short 24-48 hour cleanse is completely optional and is most recommended for those intermediate to advanced "gut healers" [individuals who have already been actively trying to heal their gut for awhile with various "gut protocols" (like GAPS, SIBO, SCD, etc.) and could benefit from a change from their norm].

Unlike traditional cleanses, you can still eat some *real* foods during this 24-48 hours, but all foods will be REALLY easy to digest, low FODMAP foods and include things like smoothies, soups, cooked vegetables, and flaky or lightly cooked proteins. The foods for your 24-48 hour cleanse are **not much different**

from your 28-Day Reset, except there is a *greater emphasis on eating lighter with low FODMAP foods, cooked vegetables, soups and broths, and easy-digesting proteins.*

Sometimes taking a short break from harder-to-digest foods (like raw veggies, cruciferous veggies, high-fructose fruit, nuts and seeds, or coffee) that certainly are "healthy foods," can be "eye opening" for some people. Even though these foods are healthy, they may not be healthy for your body (or gut) right now.

Here's the basic run down:

24-48 Hour Cleanse Protocol (Optional)

24-48 Hour Cleanse Key Points:

-Start the day off with:
- 12-16 oz. Warm Lemon Water
-8-12 oz. Celery Juice (on an empty stomach), 20-30 minutes before eating

-Eat 3 balanced meals* consisting of:
-Lean, easy-to-digest protein
-Green Veggie (cooked or raw)
-1-2 Healthy fats
-Additional Veggie (optional)
-Add 1 tbsp. Apple cider vinegar to water & consume with meals

-Eat 1 condiment-sized servings of a fermented food with a meal or as a snack

-Drink herbal tea or a cup of bone broth before bed in the evening

---

*Make one of your daily meals a soup or smoothie based meal (See Sample Meal Ideas)

Q. What About Snacks?

-During your 24-48 Hour Cleanse, consume 1-2 snacks (only if needed). Choose from the following options:
- Fresh fruit (see food list)
- Bone Broth
- Coconut Butter or Coconut Yogurt
- Fermented Vegetables
- Raw, Soaked Seeds
- Simple Vegetable Juice (no added sugar)
- Herbal Tea with Collagen

24-48 Hour "Cleanse" Food List

Consume

Easy-to-Digest Proteins
- Flaky Wild-Caught Fish
- Organic Chicken & Turkey (Shredded, Broiled, Pulled)
- Crockpot Stewed Meats (Beef, Bison, Chicken)

Cooked, Roasted & Steamed Veggies (Minimal raw leafy greens, herbs and cucumber ok)
- Sauteed or Steamed Leafy Greens (cook in coconut oil or ghee)
- Bamboo shoots
- Beet
- Bok choy
- Carrot
- Cucumber (including pickles made without sugar)
- Dandelion greens
- Endive
- Fermented vegetables (raw sauerkraut, or lactofermente vegetables)
- Fresh & dried herbs
- Green beans

- Kale (cooked)
- Lettuce
- Olives
- Parsnip
- Sea vegetables
- Spinach
- Spring onion (green part only)
- Sprouts and microgreens (including alfalfa and sunflower)
- Summer squash (zucchini, pattypan and yellow squash)
- Swiss chard
- Winter squash (acorn, butternut, pumpkin

Fruits
- Berries (Blueberries, Raspberries, Strawberries)
- Grapefruit
- Grapes
- Green Apples
- Green Tipped Banana (1/2)
- Kiwi
- Lemon/Lime
- Melon (Cantaloupe, Honeydew)
- Orange
- Papaya
- Pineapple

Healthy Fats
- Animal Fats (lard, tallow, duck fat)
- Avocado/Avocado Mayo/Avocado Oil
- Coconut (butter/flakes, oil yogurt)
- Cod liver Oil
- Ghee
- Extra Virgin Olive Oil
- Olives
- Raw seeds/seedbutter (minimal)

Fermented Foods
- Coconut Yogurt
- Kefir (Goat's Milk Kefir, Water Kefir; Not dairy)
- Kimchi
- Low-sugar kombucha
- Pickled vegetables

Avoid:
- Alcohol
- Beans, Peanuts & Soy
- Coffee
- Dairy
- Dried Fruit
- Eggs (pastured egg yolks only ok)
- Grains (Wheat, Bread, Pasta, Rice)

High FODMAP Foods (use moderation and awareness; not all FOMAPS will affect you :
- Cruciferous Veggies: Raw Kale, Brussels Sprouts, Broccoli, Cauliflower
- High Fructose Fruits: Apricots, Apples, Nectarines, Mangos, Dates, Pears, Plums, Raisins, Cherries, Watermelon, Onions
- Other High FODMAP Veggies: Artichoke, Asparagus, Leeks, Shallots

Nightshades: (Tomatoes, Tomato Paste, Chili Powder & Spices, Paprika, Curry Powder, Eggplant, Bellpeppers, Peppers)

Nuts/Nutbutter & Seeds

Pork (Slowest Digesting Meat)

Processed Powders/Bars/Packaged Goods

Sugar & Artificial Sweeteners (Including Stevia, Honey, Agave & Maple Syrup)

Vegetable Oils & High Omega 6 Fats (Canola Oil, Crisco, sunflower, safflower, grape seed,
soybean, cottonseed and peanut Oil)

The 28 Day Gut Kickstart

Sample 48-Hour "Cleanse" Menu:

Day 1
Pre-Breakfast:
12-16 oz. Warm Lemon Water
Celery Juice

Breakfast
Leftover Wild-Caught Salmon
Steamed Broccoli
Coconut Flakes

Lunch
Chicken Salad (Shredded Chicken + Avocado Mayo)
Leftover Rainbow Carrots
Pickled Cucumber
Mixed Dark Leafy Greens
Fresh Squeezed Lemon

Snack
1/2 Green Apple
Dinner
Chicken or Shredded Grass-fed Beef + Vegetable Bone Broth Soup
Post Dinner:
Herbal Tea

Day 2
Pre-Breakfast:
12-16 oz. Warm Lemon Water

Breakfast:
Breakfast Porridge (1/2 cup cooked butternut squash + 1/2 cup full fat organic coconut milk + 1 pinch salt & cinnamon + ½ green-tipped banana + toasted coconut + collagen)

Lunch: Leftover Salmon, Avocado Mayo, Olives, Mixed Greens with fresh squeezed lemon, 4 oz. Low-Sugar Kombucha

Snack: Cold Pressed Green Juice (lemon as sweetener), Turkey Jerky

Dinner: Chicken & Vegetable Soup, Avocado

Post Dinner: Herbal Tea

Assessments

In order to know where you're going (or why you may want to go somewhere else) you must know where you're coming from. *How do you feel?*

Assessment and Evaluation are crucial first components to any gut-healing protocol, essentially so you recognize your own unique gut issues—and triggers—which contribute to imbalances.

Assessment doesn't just include "blood and guts" labs either. The Gut Kickstart takes a "minimalistic" approach to both assessment and healing.

Your Gut Kickstart Assessments include:
1. Chronicle Your Personal "Gut" Timeline
2. Self-Assessment
3. Keep a 3-Day Food & Poo Log

We will also review potential labs that may be beneficial, but these 3 primary Assessments are your baseline for knowing who you are and where you're coming from in your health.

So How Do You Feel?
Find a quiet place to sit still for one minute. Close your eyes. Practice that deep, nose-based and belly breathing. And check in with your body.

Do you hear it?

How do you feel, right now, in this moment?

Stomach settled and calm? Uncomfortable or irritated?
Slightly lightheaded—it's been a minute since you ate something?
Dry mouth?
Tight muscles?
Energized? Depleted from 6 hours of sleep last night?

Calm and peace?
Refreshed?

In our go-go-go world, it's easy to **disconnect with our body** and how we feel, much less connect with how we feel in our gut health and how food makes us feel.

The number one question you will come back to time and time again throughout your 28 Day Gut Kickstart is asking your body:

How do you feel?

Nourished? Energetic? Alive? Like a baby who just did the "doo" and can now stop crying from its gassy, bloated, upset tummy? Satiated?

Or, do you feel lethargic and sluggish? Bloated? Gassy? Pimply? Constipated? Headaches? Brain foggy? Anxious? Light-headed? Fixated more on food? Depleted?

All good health, starts with digestion.

You are what you *digest*—and if or when your digestion is off, many of the signs and symptoms we've previously discussed may occur (*even* when you eat "healthy").

Assessment 1: Gut Health Timeline

Create a "Gut Health Timeline" for yourself with the top 10 events, memories and/or stressors you have in your own general health journey which may have shaped how you feel today.

List any of the top 10 stressors, events, lifestyle factors or indicators you can point back to your own gut dysfunction or health imbalances.

Some examples you may find yourself including could be:
- The first time you remember having a gut issue (like having to run out of your grade school classroom to use the bathroom or letting one "rip" during reading circle and everyone laughing)

- Taking several rounds of antibiotics for strep throat, ear infections, allergies and everything in between
- Growing up on Lunchables, Goldfish crackers, and Hamburger Helper
- Any chronic acne breakouts you had as a teen or young adult
- Trying out a specific diet plan that felt good...at first. Then left you constipated or bloated all the time
- Years of chronic constipation during college—living off Lean Cuisines, energy drinks, and protein bars
- Shoulder surgery or car wreck injury, along with the pain meds you had to take which killed off gut bacteria
- Your trip to Thailand and coming back with a tummy that didn't feel "right."

To help jog your memory, consider how any of these stressors have contributed to your health imbalances:

Physical & Lifestyle Stressors

- Blue light screen exposure (long time on screens)
- Light at night time
- Less than 7 hours of sleep most nights
- Overtraining
- Sedentary lifestyle
- Imbalanced exercise (i.e. doing HIIT or chronic cardio all the time without mixing it up)
- Exposure to chemicals in beauty, cleaning and hygiene products
- Plastic Tupperware/container use and other environmental toxins
- Mold exposure
- Lack of outdoor/nature and fresh air
- Endlessly Google searching answers to your health questions

- NSAID use (headaches, etc.)
- Oral birth control
- Long-term prescription medication use
- High coffee/caffeine consumption (more than one cup of quality coffee per day)
- Disrupted circadian rhythms for sleeping, eating, working and resting patterns
- Artificial sweeteners (most commercial stevia included)
- Eating packaged, refined or processed foods
- Low water intake (less than half your bodyweight in ounces)
- Tap water (not filtered)
- High alcohol consumption or smoking
- Frequent eating out (more than preparing/handling your food)
- Stress over food/diet
- Under-eating
- Low fiber (Fermentable prebiotic fiber foods)
- Lack of quality protein (amino acids for your brain)
- Conventional meat and dairy consumption
- Grains and "gluten free" processed products (with gluten cross-contamination)
- Binging/Purging and disordered eating habits
- Jet lag/Foreign travel
- Shift work
- Pain (joint, musculoskeletal)
- Infectious/bacterial disease
- Gut inflammation & Underlying gut conditions (SIBO, parasites, etc.)

Mental Stressors

- Type A personality
- Difficulty listening to your body over your schedule
- Relationship stress

- Financial stress/pressures
- Lack of control
- Burnout
- Not talking about your stress (bottling it up)
- Lack of play/fun
- Not doing things you love
- Serotonin suppression ("feel good" brain chemicals)
- Social media comparison/endless scrolling
- Trying to be all things to all people/people pleasing
- FOMO (lack of downtime for yourself)
- Burning a candle at both ends
- News binging
- Disconnected from community/meaningful relationships

Assessment 2: Self-Assessment

Signs & Symptoms

For each of these symptoms, rate how often and to what degree you experience the following symptoms.

never	0
rarely	1
times per month or every so often	1-2
occasionally: weekly	2
frequently/daily	3

adapted from "Signs and Symptoms Analysis from a Functional Perspective" by Dicken Weatherby

Upper GI
Belching, bloating or gas within one hour of eating
Heartburn or acid reflux
Bad breath (halitosis)
Loss of taste for meat
Strong odor in sweat
Sense of excess fullness after meals
Stomach upset by taking vitamins
Sleepy after meals

Diarrhea, chronic or after meals
Undigested food in stools
Fingernails chip, peel or break easily
Feel like skipping breakfast
Anemia, unresponsive to iron
Stomach pains or cramps
Feel better if you don't eat
Vegan diet

Small Intestine
Dairy sensitivity
Foods you could not give up
Food allergies
Airborne allergies
Crave bread or noodles or starchy carbs and fruits
Alternating constipation or diarrhea

Wheat or grain sensitivity
Pulse speeds up after eating
Feel spacey
Get hives
Sinus congestion/stuffy head
Bizarre, vivid dreams/nightmares
Use over-the-counter meds

Large Intestine
Anus itch
Stools are not well-formed
Mucus in stool
Foul smelling lower bowel gas
Dark circles under eyes
Cramping in lower abdomen
Stools are hard or difficult to pass

Feel worse in moldy place
Coated tongue
Bad breath or strong body odors
Irritable bowel or mucus colitis
Stools have corners or edges that are flattened or ribbon shaped

Less than one bowel movement per day
Fungus or yeast infections
Taken an antibiotic for a long period of time (0=never, 1=less than one months, 2=less than 3 months, 3=greater than 3 months)

Painful to press long outside of thighs (IT Band)
History of parasites (0=no, 1=yes)
Ringworm, jock itch, athlete's foot or nail fungus

Liver/Gallbladder

Pain between shoulder blades
Sensitive to chemicals (perfume, cleaning agents)
History of drug/alcohol use
Dry skin, itchy feet or skin peels on feet
Motion sickness
Nausea
Greasy or shiny stools
Stomach easily upset by fats
Bitter taste in mouth after meals
Light, clay colored stools
Chronic fatigue or Fibromyalgia
Nutrasweet (aspartame) consumption

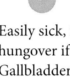

Easily sick, intoxicated or hungover if you drink wine
Gallbladder attacks
Headache over eyes
Sensitive to aspartame
Exposure to diesel fumes
Pain under right side of rib cage
History of hepatitis
Long term prescription/recreational drug use
Recovering alcohol
Alcohol per week (0=less than 3, 1= less than 7, 2=less than 14, 3=greater than 14)

Mineral Needs

History of carpal tunnel (0=no, 1=yes)
History of lower right abdominal pains or ileocecal valve problems (0=no, 1=yes)

Muscle cramps at rest
History of stress fractures or bone loss
Bursitis/Tendonitis
Clicking or popping joints

History of stress fracture
(0=no, 1=yes)
Bone loss on a bone scale
(0=no, 1=yes)
Herniated disc (0=no, 1=yes)
Morning stiffness
Crave chocolate
History of anemia
Hoarseness
Lump in throat
Difficulty swallowing/dry mouth and/or nose
Cold sores/fever blisters
Frequent skin rashes

Swelling joints
Gag easily
Lump in throat
Dry mouth/eyes/nose
White of eyes is blue tinted
Cuts heal slowly or scar easily
Decreased sense of taste or smell
White spots on fingernails
Difficulty swallowing
Morning stiffness
History of bone spurs
Feet have a strong odor

Essential Fatty Acid Deficiencies

Experience pain relief with aspirin
Crave fatty or greasy food
Tension headaches
Tension at the base of the skull

Headaches when out in the sun
Muscles easily fatigued
Low-or reduced-fat diet (current or history)
Sunburn easily
Dry, flaky skin or dandruff

Sugar Handling

Awaken a few hours after falling asleep
Crave sweets
Binge or uncontrolled appetite
Sleepy in afternoon
Crave coffee or sugar
Fatigue that is relieved by eating

Frequent thirst or urination
Family with diabetes
Shaky if meals are delayed
Irritable before meals
A headache is meals are skipped

Vitamin Deficiencies

Racing heart
Depressed
Muscles easily fatigued
Feel sore after moderate exercise
Pulse below 65 beats per minute
Ringing in ears
Numbness or tingling in hands/feet
Worrier or anxious
Night sweats
Restless leg syndrome
Nose bleeds/easily bruise
Small bumps on back of arms
MSG sensitivity
Bleeding gums when brushing teeth
Cracks at corners of mouth
Pulse below 65 beats per minute
Whole body limb jerk as falling asleep
Polyps or warts
Can hear heartbeat on pillow at night
Loss of muscle tone/heaviness in arms
Nervous or agitated
Feeling insecure
Vulnerable to insect bites

Adrenal (Stress Hormones) Imbalances

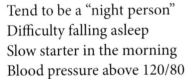

Tend to be a "night person"
Difficulty falling asleep
Slow starter in the morning
Blood pressure above 120/80
Anxiety
Headache after exercise
Clench or grind teeth
Feel wired or jittery after drinking coffee
Become dizzy when standing up suddenly
Chronic fatigue
Sweat easily
Crave salty foods
Arthritic tendencies
Allergies
Weakness, dizziness
Tendency to sprain ankles/shin splints
Afternoon yawning/headache
Salt foods before tasting
Chronic low back pain
Calm on the outside, troubled on the inside
Pain after manipulative correction
Perspire easily
Pain on medial or inner side of knee
Difficulty maintaining manipulative correction

Thyroid

Difficulty gaining or losing weight (one or the other)
Constipation
Seasonal sadness
Loss of lateral 1/3 of eyebrow
Excessive hair loss
Mentally sluggish
Easily fatigued
Fast pulse at rest
Inward trembling
Nervous, emotional
Difficulty working under pressure
Sensitive/allergic to iodine
Seasonal sadness
Reduced initiative
Sensitive to cold/poor circulation in hands or feet
Nervous or emotional/can't work under pressure
Intolerance to high temperatures
Flush easily

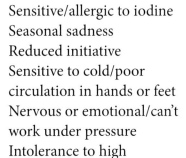

Hormonal Imbalance

Depression during periods
Mood swings associated with period (PMS)
Crave chocolate during periods
Breast tenderness with cycle
Excessive menstrual flow
Scanty blood flow during periods
Occasional skipped periods
Variations in menstrual cycles
Endometriosis
Uterine fibroids
Breast fibroids
Pain with intercourse
Vaginal discharge
Vaginal dryness
Vaginal itching
Gain weight around hips, thighs and buttocks
Excess facial or body hair
Hot flashes
Night sweats (in menopausal females)
Thinning skin

Immune System

Runny, drippy nose
Catch colds at the beginning of winter
A mucus cough
Acne
Itchy Skin
Never get sick (0=sick only 1-2 times in last 2 years, 1=not sick in last 2 years, 2=not sick in last 4 years, 3=not sick in last 7 year)
Other infections (sinus, ear, lung, skin, bladder, kidney, etc.)
Frequent colds/flu
Cysts, boils or rashes
History of Epstein Barr, Mono, Herpes, Shingles, Chronic Fatigue Syndrome, Hepatitis, or other chronic viral condition (0=no, 1=yes, in the past, 2=currently a mild condition, 3=severe)

Scoring

Add up your numbers in each section.

0-8= Low priority
9-13= Moderate Priority
14-19+=High Priority

High Priority areas point to the regions of your body most sensitive to imbalance. This screening tool can help you and/or your practitioner understand a clearer picture of where to start with lab testing or deeper digging.

Assessment 3: Keep a 3-Day Food & Poo Log

You will increase your awareness about how food makes you feel physically, mentally and emotionally by keeping track for three days, logging how you feel before and after meals (i.e., headaches, shaky, obsessing over calories, etc.). There is no need to track calories or macronutrients. We're more concerned with how you FEEL.

Also, you'll keep a 3-Day Poo Log (noting the time, shape, and texture of your poo). Check out the stool chart below for a gauge of ideal poo, as well as constipation or "transit" test you can do as a bonus!

Poo Log: Stool Assessment & Transit Time

Part 1: Stool Assessment

What does your poo say about you?

When our poop is "off," it indicates something else is "off."

Track your poo for the next three days, by simply monitoring and logging the time you go and what your poo looks like, as well as any symptoms around your potty time (i.e., bloating, cramping, stress, etc.). Use the following descriptions and the Bristol Stool Chart for guidance in assessing and achieving the "golden poo."

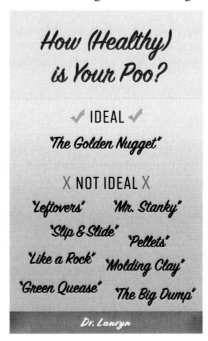

Ideal: The Golden Nugget: Medium brown. Solidly formed in the shape of an S or C. Passing 1-3 times per day.

The following poo patterns are not ideal, and while okay on occasion, if these are regularly occurring, something is off with your poo, gut health and/or food.

Leftovers. Can you see those Brussels sprouts, sweet potato or mushrooms you ate—and are still not completely broken down? This is not ideal. This shows it did not pass through the entire process of digestion. Consider your food chewing practices.

Slip & Slide. Watery and loose. Often, you can see the foods you ate in this one, too—semi-broken down. Watery stools usually mean you ate something that your body yells, "Mayday, mayday! I don't like this." A higher incidence of increased "bad" bacteria is indicated and/or food intolerances.

Green Quease. Green poo often with queasy feelings. This may indicate your gallbladder is not thoroughly breaking down bile salts to move your poop over to that brown color. Green poop is often provoked when we eat fattier foods, since bile helps break down fats, too—like vegetable oils (canola, Crisco, processed olive oil) from restaurants, processed and greasy foods (Chinese takeout, a fast food burger or greasy slice of pizza), and even "healthy" fats (like coconut oil, butter, etc.).

Molding Clay. If your stools are pale or clay-colored, you may have a problem with the drainage of your biliary system, which is comprised of your gallbladder, liver, and pancreas (similar to the Green Quease). Bile salts are released into your stools by your liver, giving the stools a brown color.

Mr. Stanky. Dark, foul, sometimes greasy and/or stinky. Something is toxic (i.e., not right). Common toxic triggers include Processed and refined foods. High amounts of non-organic, non-fresh foods and triggers. General toxicity overload. Additives and chemicals. Poor lifestyle habits (smoking, sedentary, fast food). Use of plastics.

The Big Dump. After a day or two (or three!) of not going, you finally go...all at once. You wonder: How was that in there?! You struggle with constipation and moving bowels through, until it finally decides to come and dump, leaving you feeling cleansed. May indicate low stomach acid, sluggish motility and/or bacterial overgrowth.

Like a Rock. Difficult to pass or rock-like. You still get it out—but a little straining was included. Drink more water and make sure you're eating your veggies—and the kinds your body likes (you may be eating lots of raw veggies for instance—which are harder to break down, or sensitive to FODMAPS—like broccoli and Brussels sprouts. Leafy greens—cooked down and sauteed—can be good for hard stools). Also, assess the quality of your proteins and other foods (have you been eating processed meats or packaged food items—even "paleo" bars and crackers and bread?), as well as your fat intake—are you eating fats with your meals to help lubricate your digestive tract? Sometimes your body just needs some good ol' meat, veggies and healthy fats—and plenty of water—along with time to breathe, chew and enjoy your meals (not on the go).

Pellets. Like acorns or little rocks, these come out in bits and pieces—in one sitting or throughout the day. Hard to pass and generally darker in color. Stress, low water intake, eating on the go, low fiber intake, low stomach acid and bacteria

> imbalance (low "good bacteria") all play leading roles in pellet poop. If you've experienced this, you're often thankful for whatever the poop gods will give you—but look to lifestyle factors to dig deeper and bring things up to speed with: apple cider vinegar in water before meals, prebiotic and probiotic foods, some starchy veggies and plenty of greens, chewing your food and slowing down to breathe at meals, yoga, and meditation—just to name a few.

Bonus: Poo Transit Time Test

In addition to tracking to your stool for three days, you are also going to track your transit time. How efficient is your digestion? For this test, measure the "transit time" (i.e., the time it takes for food to pass from one end to the other). Optimal transit time is considered to be 12 to 48 hours. Longer than 72 hours indicates constipation and the possibility of other gut pathologies.

How to Do It

Choose one of the following foods:

- **Sesame seeds** (one teaspoon to a tablespoon, mixed into a glass of water and swallowed whole)
- **Corn kernels** (a cup of cooked kernels eaten alone, at least an hour apart from other foods)
- **Red beets** (a cup of cooked, or raw and shredded, and eaten alone)

Whichever you choose, simply note the time you eat it, and then watch and wait for when it "reappears" in a bowel movement! Sesame seeds or corn are easy to spot, and beets give your stool a distinct purple-red color.

Bonus: At Home DIY Gut Tests

Here are a few other at-home gut health tests you can run on yourself, though the best one is still the elimination test. Positive markers on these tests can point to underlying Gut imbalances.

Stomach Acid Levels: The Apple Cider Vinegar Challenge

How is your stomach acid production?
Gauge how you feel when you take apple cider vinegar.

Stir 1-2 tablespoons of apple cider vinegar in 4 ounces of water and drink before meals. Gauge if you feel a warming sensation when consumed (a sign of increased stomach acid and digestive support). Also reflect how you generally feel digestively: Less bloating? Discomfort? The same? No change?

If you notice you feel better or less bloating, brain fog or low energy throughout the day, chances are there was a stomach acid deficiency present.

Or Try the HCL Supplement Challenge instead.
HCL or hydrochloric acid is the same type of stomach acid you have in your gut.

Take one hydrochloric acid supplement (600-700 mg with Betaine & Pepsin in the formula) with water and gradually increase the dose until you feel a burning sensation. Once burning is attained, experiment with then reducing that "burning" dose to the dose you were at just prior to that burning sensation and taking supplements with meals. Note how you feel.

Do not do the HCL supplement challenge if pregnant, or frequently taking PPI, steroid drugs or NSAIDs.

Elimination Testing

If you suspect a food intolerance, the easiest way to test yourself is to simply try eliminating the trigger food from your diet altogether for at least 3 to 7 days. Note how you feel. Better? Symptom free? No change? After your time is up, reintroduce it with a meal and…just see. How do you feel now? Did any symptoms return?

If that's not it, then it may be something else like a different trigger food, the quality of the food (organic vs. non organic), a lack of digestive health and support, stress—or any combination of these.

Note: *For most accurate results with the food elimination test, eliminate and test just one food—as opposed to multiple foods—at a time.*

Bacterial Imbalance: Carbohydrate Malabsorption

Do you have bacterial imbalance ("dysbiosis"), Candida or SIBO (small intestinal bacterial overgrowth)?

Breath testing and stool testing are the most common laboratory testing measures to assess bacterial imbalances and underlying gut conditions. **However,** the Carbohydrate Malabsorption Test is an excellent DIY at home test to assess for common signs that something may not be right with your gut bacteria.

Carbohydrates (particularly starches and FODMAP foods, like apples, broccoli and onions), contain sugars which require special enzymes in your gut and saliva to break down. And in those with SIBO or Candida, the overgrown bacteria easily feeds on the unabsorbed starch and other carbs. The result? An overload of undigested starch and MORE bacteria or yeast when we eat certain starchy foods.

If you are deficient in digestive enzyme or have bacteria/yeast overgrowth, starchy foods and FODMAP foods may trigger symptoms like:

- Bloating
- Constipation
- Diarrhea/loose stools
- Blood sugar highs and lows
- Headaches/brain fog
- Skin breakouts
- Feeling sleepy after eating

The Carbohydrate Malabsorption Test is a food experiment and self-monitoring log to assess if certain carbohydrate foods trigger symptoms common in bacterial imbalance and leaky gut.

How to Do It

Step 1: Select one carbohydrate to test from the "Carbohydrate Malabsorption Test List" (below). Start with just one.

Step 2: Gradually incorporate the starch of choice into your diet over the course of three or four days, in the following example sequence:

- **Day 1** – 1/2 cup of mashed sweet potato (or other starch of choice, eaten alone)
- **Day 2** – 1/2 cup of mashed sweet potato at breakfast or lunch and 1/2 cup at dinner
- **Day 3** – ¾- 1 cup at breakfast or lunch and ¾- 1 cup at dinner
- **Day 4 (optional)** – 1/2 cup with healthy fat (like coconut butter, grass-fed butter, coconut oil) at lunch and/or dinner

Step 3: Track It. Keep a food log over your three-day experiment to note how you feel. You can use the same log you use to monitor your poo and other foods. Record not only what you eat, but how you feel before and after meals. Do you feel bloated? Gassy?

Loose stools? These foods are NOT "bad," but can point to signs that bacteria is having a "heyday" inside.

Step 4: If bloating, fatigue, blood sugar highs and lows, constipation, heartburn, skin flares, allergy flares, or other GI distress is indicated, carbohydrate malabsorption may be at play.

Carbohydrate Malabsorption Test List

Note: Each type of starch is its own food. You might do just fine with sweet potatoes but not rice. Each type of starch-containing food needs to be evaluated independently.

- Sweet Potatoes
- Rice
- Parsnips
- Potatoes
- Yuca
- Taro
- Tapioca (Cassava)
- Plantains
- Rutabaga
- Beans/Legumes

Nutrient Deficiencies: Leaky Gut

Check to see if any of the following sound familiar. If you answer yes to more than 3 items from this list, malabsorption, low stomach acid and/or underlying gut pathologies could be at play.

- White spots on fingernails
- Dark circles under eyes
- Polyps or warts regularly
- Cracks on lips or corners of mouth
- Bleeding gums, especially when brushing teeth
- Crave salty or sweet foods

- Arthritic tendencies, stiff or popping joints.
- Small bumps on backs of arms or legs, or peach fuzz hair on body
- Hoarse voice
- History anemia
- Crave chocolate regularly
- Feet or sweat has a strong odor
- Muscles always tight, despite stretching or massage
- Foot, calf or muscle cramps at rest
- Catch colds, allergies or get sick easily (more than 1-2 times per year)
- Cold sores or fever blisters
- Bone loss/Osteoporosis
- Cuts heal slowly/scar easily
- Anxiety/worrier
- Whole body limb jerk before falling asleep
- Numbness/tingling in hands and feet
- Ringing in ears
- Pulse below 65 per minute
- Can hear heartbeat on pillow
- Night sweats
- Easily fatigued or sore after moderate exercise
- Catch colds, allergies or get sick easily (more than 1-2 times per year)
- Low Vitamin D diagnosis in past 12 months

How do you feel? Common Signs of Nutrient Deficiencies

Without looking too deeply into testing or assessments, sometimes your body signs are direct indicators of a gut imbalance or nutrient deficiency. Do any of these fit for you?

1. Soft or Brittle Fingernails.
What it may mean: Low Calcium.

Other Common Symptoms of Low Calcium:
- Frequent skin rashes/hives
- Muscle cramps
- Poor growth
- Bone/joint pain
- Joints pop or click
- Frequent hoarseness
- High/low blood pressure
- Easily get nosebleeds

What to Do About It:
- Take Cod Liver Oil (Vitamin A & D) + Vitamin K2 + Magnesium
- Improve gut health and absorption with HCL and digestive enzymes
- Eat calcium-rich real foods like spinach, kale, broccoli, sardines and bone-in fish, sesame seeds, almonds, full-fat organic plain dairy, basil, thyme, cumin, and dill.

Note: Calcium supplementation is rarely necessary. Often, people actually lack the co-factors which help with the uptake of calcium in the first place, including: Magnesium, Vitamin D, Vitamin K and Vitamin A.

2. Frequent Headaches
What it may mean: Blood-Sugar Imbalance, Low Water or Low Fat Intake and/or Leaky Gut (not absorbing your nutrients to nourish your brain)

Other Common Symptoms of Blood Sugar Imbalance:
- Sugar cravings

- Caffeine cravings
- Binge/uncontrolled eating
- Irritable before meals
- Shaky if meals are delayed
- Frequent thirst or urination
- Fatigue relieved by eating or drinking coffee
- Awaken shortly after going to sleep
- Excessive appetite
- Low fat intake

What to Do About It:
- Eat healthy fats and protein with meals and snacks.
- Increase meal time portions if you aren't eating enough.
- Increase water intake, and start day off with a glass of warm lemon water + sea salt
- Incorporate healthy exercise into your day
- Wean off coffee with Teeccino herbal tea (tastes like coffee), herbal tea, and "bulletproof" Chai (add butter/MCT oil to Chai)

3. Adult Acne/Skin Breakouts
What it may mean: Low Stomach Acid

Skin breakouts indicate your body is not fully absorbing the foods you're feeding it, and/or you're not feeding it the balanced real foods it needs in the first place. (Our skin eats what we eat and absorb).

Other Common Symptoms of Low Stomach Acid:
- Bloating after meals
- Belching/gas within an hour of eating
- Feel better if you don't eat
- Sleepy after meals
- Undigested food in stools

- Stomach pains or cramps
- Dysbiosis (bacterial imbalance)
- Loss of taste for meat
- Bad breath

What to Do About It:
- Add 1 tablespoon of apple cider vinegar to water (2-4 oz.) before meals
- Chew your food
- Slow down when you eat
- Take an HCL supplement
- Add beet juice or beets to your food routine
- Drink water throughout the day
- Incorporate fermented foods and/or a probiotic into your daily supplement routine
- Exercise—but don't over-do it

4. Upset Stomach after Eating Red Meat or Fats (even Healthy Fats)
What it may mean: Gallbladder Dysfunction
Your gallbladder helps break down fats. "Biliary stasis" can happen in the gallbladder with low-fat or low-fiber diets, low water intake, stress, and high consumption of vegetable oils and processed foods.

Other Common Symptoms of Gallbladder Dysfunction:
- Light or clay colored stool
- Greasy or shiny stools
- Pain between shoulder blades
- Gallbladder attacks
- Nausea
- History of morning sickness
- Motion sickness

What to Do About It:
- Incorporate beets into your daily diet or smoothies
- Herbs which cleanse the liver
- Taking an HCL supplement to improve digestion (yes, back to the gut)
- Eat greens and veggies with your healthy fats and proteins
- Cut out processed foods and vegetable oils (canola, soy, grape-seed, Crisco)
- Take a liver/gall-bladder support (like Ox Bile or Beta TCP by Biotics Research)

5. Dry Flaky Skin
What it may mean: Essential Fatty Acid Insufficiency
If you're using lotion frequently to moisturize your skin, it may mean a fatty-acid insufficiency is present also due to "biliary dysfunction" (as discussed above)—leading to incomplete breakdown and absorption of healthy fats.

Other Common Symptoms of Essential Fatty Acid Insufficiency:
- Pain relieved with aspirin for random pains
- Muscles easily fatigued
- Headaches when out in hot sun
- Tension headaches at base of skull
- Crave fatty or greasy foods
- Mineral deficiency (especially Zinc)

What to Do About It:
- Find a healthy fat supplement for you (flaxseed oil, EPA/DHA from fish oil, blackcurrant seed oil)
- Incorporate fatty fish (wild-caught) 1-2 times per week
- Consider an HCL supplement, probiotic, and/or digestive enzymes to improve digestion

- Incorporate beets into your daily diet or smoothies
- Eat greens and veggies with your healthy fats to increase absorption
- Cut out processed foods and vegetable oils (canola, soy, grape-seed, Crisco)
- Don't fear the fat

6. Tired—Even if You Slept 8 Hours

What it may mean: B12 Deficiency or Subclinical Hypothyroidism/Thyroid Dysfunction

Other Common Symptoms of B12 Deficiency:
- You can barely stay awake in the afternoon—even if you slept eight hours
- Numbness & tingling in extremities
- Muscles easily fatigued
- Forgetfulness
- Dizzy or wobbly when you stand up
- Pale skin
- Smooth red tongue (losing the papillae—those little bumps—on your tongue)
- Easily stressed/anxious
- Blurred vision or spots of light

Other Common Symptoms of Thyroid Dysfunction:
- Stubborn weight gain, unexplained weight loss or a "stuck" metabolism
- Loss of desire
- Brittle fingernails
- Dull hair
- Low energy

What to Do About It:

- Address underlying factors (digestion, environmental toxins, blood sugar regulation)
- Take an HCL supplement and/or digestive enzymes to improve digestion (yes, back to the gut)
- Take a Vitamin B12 supplement or B-Complex
- Include a whole-sourced protein, fat, and green veggies with each meal
- Take cod liver oil
- Take a zinc supplement (if low in zinc) or eat organ meats and shellfish
- Add iodine to your diet (Use Kelp granules on vegetables—like salt, Iodized salt, Kelp, Sea Vegetables and Seafood)

Assessment 4: Lab Assessments (Optional)

Beyond at-home DIY Testing, professional lab testing can be one of the most direct routes to assessing your particular gut health presentation.

The following labs are recommended as a "baseline" Gut Kickstart Testing protocol in order to "test, not guess" if any underlying conditions may be at play in your personal get health:

1. Comprehensive Stool Assessment & Parasitology (such as Doctor's Data or GI Map)
2. Complete Functional Blood Chemistry Panel

Connect with a functional medicine practitioner or healthcare professional familiar with functional lab testing. Many practitioners work with clients worldwide, so distance is not an issue.

Functional Medicine Practitioner Directories
Kresser Institute Practitioners

Institute for Functional Medicine

Functional Medicine Coaching Academy

Above all, testing allows you to "test, not guess."

The remainder of this chapter is devoted to teaching you how to interpret your lab tests and clinical assessments, including. If you have not had any lab work completed or don't plan to do so, then skip to the next chapter Phase 2: The 28 Day Reset.

Note: If you're not ready to take the leap, no sweat. The initial 28 Day Gut Kickstart protocol is the BEST place to start, especially if you're new to an anti-inflammatory diet. Removing the top inflammatory foods for an initial 28 days will best allow you to test and see if your gut symptoms are more related to your diet or actual gut health itself.

Overview of Lab Tests & Assessments

The following is an overview of several gut assessments and tests you may run—either at home or a practitioner's office, as well as a cheat sheet for determining which test is best for you (if any), depending on your symptoms.

Lab Tests & Assessments Overview

Complete Functional Blood Chemistry Panel
Food Intolerance Testing
Autoimmune Condition Testing
SIBO Breath Testing
OATS (Organic Acids Testing)
Intestinal Permeability Testing
Stool Testing
GI Scope

Complete Functional Blood Chemistry Panel

A serum blood chemistry panel is the classic "gold" standard when it comes to any traditional doctor's visit. Blood work *can* be beneficial for seeing some nutrient deficiencies and body imbalances.

Unfortunately though, most traditional blood lab work runs into two problems:

1.) Blood Work Doesn't Consider Gut Health. Traditional Blood work catches nutrient deficiencies by assessing for nutrients and minerals like Vitamin D, Iron, Calcium and Magnesium levels. If they are low, often your doctor will prescribe a supplement, medication or certain foods to address the issue. However, if you are UNABLE to digest those nutrients in the first place, *then* you still won't digest the supplements or nutrients you're taking, or those nutrients MAY not be the nutrient you need in the first place (for example: low calcium is usually an indicator you are missing out on calcium **cofactors** like Vitamin D, Vitamin A, or magnesium—not calcium itself, and supplementing with too much calcium can actually be detrimental to your heart health).

2.) Traditional Blood Work Tests for Disease, NOT Disease Prevention. Blood panel lab results contain a "normal lab range" value they want your blood numbers to fall into for each marker (for example: A healthy thyroid TSH lab range is 0.5 to 4.5). If your results fall out of that range, your doctor tells you that you are "unhealthy" or in a **diseased state.**

However, traditional blood work lab ranges FAIL to detect imbalances or potential problems BEFORE they become a problem (i.e. the PREVENTION of disease).

Enter: a functional blood chemistry lab panel—lab ranges which are typically a little bit narrower to identify diseases or imbalances before they occur to the fullest.

Back to the TSH thyroid lab test for instance: The standard lab range for testing thyroid-stimulating hormone, or TSH, is typically 0.5 to 4.5, **but** the functional range is 0.5 to 2.5 or even 2. Often times when a person's TSH is **above** 2.5, they begin experiencing symptoms of thyroid dysfunction (such as unwanted weight gain, constipation, bloating, fatigue, etc.)

Hence, the functional lab range allows you and your clinician to address thyroid health **before** it gets to a full-blown thyroid condition, like hypothyroidism.

The bottom line?
Most standard lab range values test your blood to catch disease when disease is ALREADY present.

Functional blood chemistry labs, on the other hand, help catch disease (as well as nutrient imbalances and gut health markers) before it's at a full-blown disease state.

What to do about it?
Connect with a functional medicine trained practitioner who is familiar with functional blood chemistry for a better picture of your body's true imbalances and needs.

What are some ranges I should be aware of for gut health on a blood panel?
Any signs of nutrient imbalances and deficiencies typically point back to a gut imbalance and dietary deficiency. Again, if you are NOT absorbing or digesting your food or supplements in the

first place, then of course you are going to have an "off" lab value on a blood test.

Here are some functional lab ranges (compared to standard lab ranges) for common markers and symptoms tested to keep in mind for assessing your own gut health on your blood panel (remember to look at the functional lab ranges as your personal "gold standard").

If you notice these patterns of being high or low, this may indicate an imbalance:

Impaired liver function *Common Symptoms*:
   Motion Sickness
   Nausea
   Light or Clay Colored Stools
   Pain Under Right Side of Rib Cage
   Fibromyalgia
   Gallbladder Attacks

AST (high)	**Functional Lab Range: 0-25**	**Standard Lab Range: 0-40**
ALT (high)	**Functional Lab Range:** 0-26	**Standard Lab Range:** 0-44
GGT (high)	**Functional Lab Range:** 0-29	**Standard Lab Range:** 0-65
LDH (high)	**Functional Lab Range:** 140–180	**Standard Lab Range:** 120-225
Alkaline phosphatase (high)	**Functional Lab Range:** 42–107	**Standard Lab Range:** 39–117

Impaired gallbladder function *Common Symptoms*:
- Motion Sickness
- Nausea
- Light or Clay Colored Stools
- Pain Under Right Side of Rib Cage
- Fibromyalgia + Gallbladder Attacks

GGT (high)	**Functional Lab Range:** 0-29	**Standard Lab Range:** 0-65
ALT (high)	**Functional Lab Range:** 0-26	**Standard Lab Range:** 0-44
AST (high)	**Functional Lab Range:** 0-25	**Standard Lab Range:** 0-40
Bilirubin (high)	**Functional Lab Range:** 0.1-1.2	**Standard Lab Range:** 1.1-2.5
Alkaline phosphatase (high)	**Functional Lab Range:** 42-107	**Standard Lab Range:** None
LDH (high)	**Functional Lab Range:** 140–180	**Standard Lab Range:** 120-225

Thyroid Hypofunction *Common Symptoms*:
Constipation
Unwanted Weight Gain

TSH (high)	**Functional Lab Range:** 0.5-2.0	**Standard Lab Range:** 0.450-4.50
T4, total (low)	**Functional Lab Range:** 6-12	**Standard Lab Range:** 4.5-12
T3, total (low)	**Functional Lab Range:** 100-180	**Standard Lab Range:** 70-180
Free thyroxine index (low)	**Functional Lab Range:** 0-3	**Standard Lab Range:** None

T3, free (low)	**Functional Lab Range:** 2.5-4.0	**Standard Lab Range:** 2-4.5
T4, free (low)	**Functional Lab Range:** 1.0-1.5	**Standard Lab Range:** 0.8-1.77
Reverse T3 (high)	**Functional Lab Range:** 9-21	**Standard Lab Range:** 9.2-24
TPO antibodies (high)	**Functional Lab Range:** 0-34	**Standard Lab Range:** 0-34
TG antibodies (high)	**Functional Lab Range:** 0-0.9	**Standard Lab Range:** 0-0.9

Thyroid Hyperfunction *Common Symptoms*:
    Constipation
    Unwanted Weight Loss
    Fatigue

TSH (low)	**Functional Lab Range:** 0.5-2.0	**Standard Lab Range:** 0.450-4.50
T4, total (high)	**Functional Lab Range:** 6-12	**Standard Lab Range:** 4.5-12
T3, total (high)	**Functional Lab Range:** 100-180	**Standard Lab Range:** 70-180
Free thyroxine index (high)	**Functional Lab Range:** 0-3	**Standard Lab Range:** None
T4, free (high)	**Functional Lab Range:** 1.0-1.5	**Standard Lab Range:** 0.8-1.77
T3, free (high)	**Functional Lab Range:** 2.5-4.0	**Standard Lab Range:** 2-4.5
TPO antibodies (high)	**Functional Lab Range:** 0-34	**Standard Lab Range:** 0-34
TG antibodies (high)	**Functional Lab Range:** 0-0.9	**Standard Lab Range:** 0-0.9

High Cholesterol *Common Symptoms*:
- **Inflammation**
- **Bloating**
- **Constipation**
- **Bacterial Overgrowth**
- **Leaky Gut**
- **Allergies**

Total cholesterol (high)	**Functional Lab Range:** 150-230	**Standard Lab Range:** 100-199
LDL (high)	**Functional Lab Range:** 0-140	**Standard Lab Range:** 0-99
Total Cholesterol / HDL Ratio (high)	**Functional Lab Range:** /2	**Standard Lab Range:** /3.8
HDL (low)	**Functional Lab Range:** 55-85	**Standard Lab Range:** 40+
Triglycerides (high)	**Functional Lab Range:** 50-100	**Standard Lab Range:** 0-149

B12 deficiency *Common Symptoms*:
- **Bloating**
- **Constipation**

Serum B12 (low)	**Functional Lab Range:** 450-2000	**Standard Lab Range:** 211-946
HoloTC (low)	**Functional Lab Range:** 0-3	**Standard Lab Range:** None
Serum MMA (high)	**Functional Lab Range:** 0-300	**Standard Lab Range:** 0-378
Homocysteine (high)	**Functional Lab Range:** 0-7	**Standard Lab Range:** 0-15

Parasite infection *Common Symptoms*:
- IBS-D or IBS-C
- SIBO & Bacterial Overgrowth

Eosinophils (high)	**Functional Lab Range:** 0-3	**Standard Lab Range:** None
WBC (high)	**Functional Lab Range:** 5.0-8.0	**Standard Lab Range:** 3.4-10.8
Monocytes (high)	**Functional Lab Range:** 4-7	**Standard Lab Range:** None

Inflammation *Common Symptoms*:
- **Allergies**
- **Skin Breakouts**
- **Low Immunity**
- **Constipation/Bloating**
- **Fatigue**

WBC (high)	**Functional Lab Range:** 5.0-8.0	**Standard Lab Range:** 3.4-10.8
Neutrophils (high)	**Functional Lab Range:** 40-60	**Standard Lab Range:** None
Lymphocytes (high or low)	**Functional Lab Range:** 25-40	**Standard Lab Range:** None
Ferritin (high)	**Functional Lab Range:** 30-200	**Standard Lab Range:** 30-400
CRP (high)	**Functional Lab Range:** 0-1.0	**Standard Lab Range:** 0-3.0
HDL (>85)	**Functional Lab Range:** 55-85	**Standard Lab Range:** Below 40

Magnesium deficiency *Common Symptoms*:
   Constipation

| Magnesium (<2.0) | **Functional Lab** **Range:** 2.0- 2.6 | **Standard Lab** **Range:** 1.6-2.3 |

Hyperglycemia / Met Syn (primary markers) *Common Symptoms*:
Quick Bursts of Energy—followed by crashes
Bloating
Sugar & Caffeine Cravings
Hungry or Needs Snacks Often

Fasting glucose (high)	**Functional Lab** **Range:** 75- 85	**Standard Lab** **Range:** 65-99
Hemoglobin A1c (high)	**Functional Lab** **Range:** 4.6-5.3	**Standard Lab** **Range:** 4.8-5.6
Triglycerides (high)	**Functional Lab** **Range:** Above 3	**Standard Lab** **Range:** Above 5
Triglycerides / HDL ratio (high)	**Functional Lab** **Range:** 2	**Standard Lab** **Range:** 3.8
Post-meal glucose (high)	**Functional Lab** **Range:** 75- 85	**Standard Lab** **Range:** 65-99
HDL (low)	**Functional Lab** **Range:** 55- 85	**Standard Lab** **Range:** Below 40

Hypoglycemia *Common Symptoms*:
   Blood Sugar Dips
   Sleepy when hungry
   Shaky Before Meals

| Glucose (low) | **Functional Lab** **Range:** 75- 85 | **Standard Lab** **Range:** 65-99 |

| LDH (low) | **Functional Lab Range:** 140–180 | **Standard Lab Range:** 120-225 |

Dehydration *Common Symptoms:*
- **Thirst Confused as Hunger**
- **Low Stomach Acid**
- **Bloating**
- **Constipation**

BUN (high)	**Functional Lab Range:** 8-19	**Standard Lab Range:** 8-19
Carbon Dioxide (high)	**Functional Lab Range:** 25–30	**Standard Lab Range:** 18-29
RBC (high)	**Functional Lab Range:** 4.4–4.9	**Standard Lab Range:** 4.14-5.8
Hemoglobin (high)	**Functional Lab Range:** 14–15	**Standard Lab Range:** 12-18
Hematocrit (high)	**Functional Lab Range:** 40–48	**Standard Lab Range:** 37.5-51
Sodium (high)	**Functional Lab Range:** 135–140	**Standard Lab Range:** 134-144
Potassium (low)	**Functional Lab Range:** 4–4.5	**Standard Lab Range:** 3.5-5.2

Anemia
- **Fatigue**
- **Weakness**
- **Malabsorption**
- **Low Stomach Acid**
- **Low Energy**

RBC (low)	**Functional Lab Range:** 4.4–4.9	**Standard Lab Range:** 4.14-5.8

Hemoglobin (low)	**Functional Lab Range:** 14–15	**Standard Lab Range:** 12-18
Hematocrit (low)	**Functional Lab Range:** 40–48	**Standard Lab Range:** 37.5-51
MCV (low)	**Functional Lab Range:** 85–92	**Standard Lab Range:** 79-97
MCH (low)	**Functional Lab Range:** 27–32	**Standard Lab Range:** 26-33
MCHC (low)	**Functional Lab Range:** 32–35	**Standard Lab Range:** 31.5-35.7
RDW (high)	**Functional Lab Range:** 11.5–15	**Standard Lab Range:** 12.3-15.4
Ferritin (low)	**Functional Lab Range:** 30-200	**Standard Lab Range:** 30-400
Iron (low)	**Functional Lab Range:** 40-135	**Standard Lab Range:** 40-155
Iron saturation (low)	**Functional Lab Range:** 17-45	**Standard Lab Range:** 15-55
UIBC (high)	**Functional Lab Range:** 175-350	**Standard Lab Range:** 150-375
TIBC (high)	**Functional Lab Range:** 275-425	**Standard Lab Range:** 250-450

Food Intolerance Testing

Food Intolerance and Allergy Testing are popular assessments conducted by nutritionists and doctors alike.

Food intolerance testing is ***different*** from food allergy testing.

A food allergy happens when you have an acute (sudden onset) allergic or histamine response to a food (such as hives, eyes swelling, immediate skin breakouts, swelling tissues on your tongue or mouth, trouble breathing).

A food intolerance on the other hand is a "sensitivity" that is more chronic and quieter. It manifests in signs and symptoms that you may learn to "deal with," and don't necessarily immediately impact you after you eat the food (or you may not realize they do), such as chronic fatigue, pimples, bloating, gas, constipation, seasonal allergies, and blood sugar imbalances.

Food intolerance testing tests the **antibodies** that form in your own body when you eat certain foods (like wheat, dairy, nuts, corn, fruits, etc.).

When our body forms antibodies to certain foods, an immune response occurs leading to inflammation and the body attacking itself (i.e. those side effects of gas, bloating, stomach pains, etc.).

You CAN have food intolerances *without* food allergies, and, unfortunately, the statistic of people with food intolerances goes underreported since many people blame their symptoms on the symptoms themselves (i.e. diabetes, SIBO, bloating, acne, seasonal allergies, etc.) rather than looking to underlying intolerance issues.

Food intolerance testing can help you figure out exactly what foods do and do not agree with your gut—especially if you're having a hard time deciphering it yourself during your Mindful Food Journal Assessment Phase.

Note: Not all food intolerance tests are created equal!

For starters: Many food intolerance tests on the market are NOT testing for the foods how you typically would consume them.

For instance: One food intolerance test may test your sensitivity to eggs or chicken, BUT it tests the raw antigen version forms of these food—not the cooked. Therefore the results reflected may not be 100% accurate.

Another issue many standard food intolerance tests (including ALCAT, LRA or MRT testing) run into is that they use methods of food intolerance testing that have never been clinically tested or proven.

These specific food intolerance tests involve placing a drop of your patient's blood onto a plate that's coated with a liquid or dried food extract to sit. Then, the plate is examined under a microscope every 30 minutes for up to 2 hours, depending on the test, and a technician looks for changes in the structure and shape of the white blood cells. If there are changes in the size, shape or inactivity of the cell, a "positive food intolerance" is then indicated.

In addition, since these food intolerance tests involve a technician to judge whether or not the result is "positive" leaves LOTS of room for human errors—since no two humans' interpretations will be the same.

So what test should I use?
To date, there is one lab that is testing intolerance foods you eat based on how it is typically consumed (raw vs. cooked)—Cyrex Labs.

In addition, Cyrex runs a standard blood panel sample via blood serum (as opposed to a drop of blood on a plate that is tested by a human eye).

Ask your practitioner about running one of their Array Panels to hack your own gut health:

Food Intolerance Test Suggestions:
Cyrex Array 3- Gluten & Wheat Sensitivity
Cyrex Array 4- Gluten & Wheat Cross-Reactive Foods
Cyrex Array 10- 180 Different Foods You Eat

Allergy Testing

Identifying allergies is ***different*** from testing for food intolerances.

Common allergy testing for any food (gluten, peanuts, dairy, etc.) in a doctor's office involves a "skin prick" test or blood testing.

During the skin prick test, an allergist places a drop of solution containing the food allergen on your forearm or back. Using a small plastic probe or needle, the doctor gently pricks or scratches the skin to allow a tiny amount of the solution to enter just below the surface. Results usually appear within 30 minutes. Positive results are indicated by a wheal – a raised white bump surrounded by a small circle of itchy red skin. In general, a large wheal is more likely to indicate a true food allergy, but size is not always an accurate predictor. If no wheal appears, it is unlikely that you are allergic to the test food.

As for blood testing, doctors assess for immune reactions to IgE antibodies in foods to diagnose the allergy.

However, both of these methods are still not conclusive, as approximately 50-60 percent of all blood tests and skin prick tests will yield a "false positive" result. This means that the test shows positive even though you are *NOT* allergic to the food being tested.

False allergy readings occur for two reasons:

1. **The test may be measuring your response to the *undigested* food proteins instead of an allergy to the food.**
2. **The test may detect foods that are similar among foods but do NOT trigger allergic reactions.** For example, if you are allergic to peanuts, your tests may show a positive response to other foods in the legume family, such as green beans, even if eating green beans has never been a problem for you.

So why even bother if there is at least a 50% chance of an inaccurate result?!
Exactly. For this reason food sensitivity or intolerance testing can be a clearer indicator of some potential trigger foods causing inflammation in your body, BUT the gold standard (above all) for both food allergy and food intolerance testing is within YOU and it involves an Elimination and Reintroduction protocol.

Similar to your Gut Kickstart Protocol Nutrition Blueprint—take potential trigger foods out of your diet for a short amount of time, then add them back in.

Note how you feel.

Autoimmune Condition Testing (like Celiac Disease)

There are several blood tests available which screen for celiac disease antibodies, but the most commonly used one is called a tTG-IgA test in a traditional GI doctor's office. Food intolerance testing with Cyrex Labs Array 3 panel is also an accurate way to screen for celiac and wheat/gluten sensitivities.

If this test comes back positive your physician will recommend a biopsy of your small intestine to confirm the diagnosis. A biopsy is taken from small intestine tissue and analyzed to see if there is any damage consistent with celiac disease. The diagnosis may also be confirmed when improvement is seen while on a gluten-free diet.

Note: Individuals with Celiac or high gluten sensitivities are often also intolerant or sensitive to gluten cross-contaminating foods with similar proteins as gluten, including: soy, corn, dairy, eggs, oats, barley, buckwheat, quinoa, tapioca, and instant coffee. Just because the label says "gluten free" does not mean your gut can handle it.

Coca's Pulse Food Sensitivity Test
An at-home DIY version of food sensitivity testing, the Coca's Pulse Test was designed by allergist Arthur Coca, MD as a simple

and effective way to help his patients recognize intolerances, allergies and sensitivities they may have to food.

The test is based on the fact that stress from the food(s) you are intolerant to will cause the pulse to increase. The sensory information alone from the taste buds in the mouth informs your central nervous system of the nature of the test food. If the test food is stressful to the body, there will be a short-term reaction, causing the heart to beat faster.

Although this is NOT an exact science, it can be just as accurate—if not more—than many food tests that you spend thousands of dollars on, and if anything, it is a helpful tool.

Coca's Pulse Test Procedure:
1. Conduct this test 1-2 hours after eating or drinking anything and start when you are mentally, emotionally and physically relaxed.
2. While sitting, find your pulse (with two fingers on your upper right side of your neck or either wrist) take your pulse for one full minute (don't take it for 15-30 seconds and multiply). Take a deep breath and slowly exhale. Count how many times your heart beats in one exact minute. Record this pulse rate.
3. Next, place a piece of the food in question in your mouth. It is okay to chew, but don't swallow. Taste the food for at least 30 seconds.
4. Then take your pulse again for a full minute with the food in your mouth.
5. Spit out the food and rinse your mouth with filtered water.
6. **If the pulse rate rises 6 or more points with the food in your mouth, it indicates a stress reaction** and that food should be avoided.

7. Let the pulse return to the baseline before testing with a different food.

Note: Know that the results of food sensitivity testing will also greatly depend on your mindset. If you think: "I KNOW I will be sensitive to this food!" then it will most likely sway the test results. Also, remember that food sensitivities can heal through diet and lifestyle changes, so it will be possible to re-test and reintroduce some foods after a period of gut healing.

OATS (Organic Acids Test)

Organic acids are markers of cellular metabolism, toxic exposure, nutrient imbalances, and intestinal microbial overgrowth.

Bacteria in yeast produces metabolites of small molecular weight that can appear in the urine—and sometimes there is "bad" bacteria (microbes which cause can disease and gut symptoms). The cause of high levels of acids may include oral antibiotic use, high sugar diets, immune deficiencies, acquired infections, as well as genetic factors.

The OATS test assesses over 70 different markers to determine the health of the cells in your small intestine and large intestine and any bacteria overgrowth in there.

Abnormally high levels of bacterial microorganisms in the body can cause or worsen symptoms of gut health, as well as your mental health, fatigue, and immune function (since many people with chronic illnesses, gut imbalances, or neurological disorders often excrete several abnormal organic acids in their urine).

OATS testing can also help point to the possibility of other underlying pathogens—like SIBO, dysbiosis or parasites—and help you customize the appropriate probiotics and antimicrobial supplements to take (i.e. you don't want to be taking the same bacteria you have too much of in your gut).

All you have to do? Pee in a cup that is sent to your home or at your doctor's office and send it off to the lab.

SIBO (Small Intestinal Bacterial Overgrowth) Breath Test

Small Intestinal Bacterial Overgrowth (SIBO) is an often under-diagnosed and treated problem which many people chalk up to "normal" bloating, skin breakouts, ongoing constipation, allergies, nutrient deficiencies, and/or dull/lifeless nails and hair. In fact, many people won't experience gut symptoms at all, but experience other symptoms (such as autoimmune conditions, ADD/ADHD, B12 deficiency, chronic fatigue, hormone imbalances, etc.), so very few doctors think to screen for SIBO.

If you *are* able to identify bacterial overgrowth in your gut and treat it appropriately—typically with antimicrobial herbal supplements which kill off the overgrowth of bacteria—your symptoms can improve tremendously.

Testing is typically conducted either with an endoscopy in a GI doctor's office or a breath test the patient performs at home in a home test-tube kit over the course of 2-3 hours. Since the breath test is less invasive to your gut lining, it is my preferred method of choice. The test evaluates for small intestine bacterial overgrowth (SIBO) by detecting both hydrogen and methane gas. SIBO cannot be diagnosed with a stool test or a urine test.

There are two types of breath testing: **Lactulose** or **Glucose.** During both tests, you consume a lactulose or glucose sample, then over the course of three hours, breathe into the tube every 30 minutes.

Both tests assess for SIBO by measuring the reactions of hydrogen and methane gas your body produces in response to the ingestion of "sugar" in the lactulose or glucose (what bacteria love to feed off).

If there is an abnormally high spike in the results measured from the hydrogen and methane in your test tubes at particular time intervals, then this indicates a positive reading.

While both lactulose and glucose testing assess for the amount of hydrogen spikes, lactulose breath testing gives you a bigger picture perspective of SIBO markers *throughout a greater majority of the* digestive tract (since glucose is absorbed much further up in the digestive tract than lactulose).

In short, lactulose breath testing provides the clinician with a better picture of SIBO.

SIBO breath testing is fairly straightforward and is something you can do at home with a test kit. All it requires is that you carve out about three hours one day to conduct it at home and consume the SIBO test prep diet 48 hours prior to the test.

The SIBO Test Prep Diet:
Two Days Before: Avoid all high-fiber and lactose-containing foods (i.e. dairy, whole grains, many fruits, starchy veggies, beans).

24 Hours Before: Stick to meat, fish, or poultry, plain steamed long grain white rice, eggs, and clear meat broth (no bone broth), small amounts of fat and oils, salt and pepper, water and tea.

12 Hours Before: Water fast. Avoid everything except for water. On the day of the test, be awake at least one hour prior to the test. May brush teeth, but do not smoke or do vigorous exercise.

Note: Even though SIBO breath testing is the current method of choice, it is **not** perfect, and sometimes test results can come back with a false negative due to the potential for many human errors along the way. That said, if you suspect SIBO (particularly with bloating after meals, chronic constipation or malabsorption issues present), it can often be treated *as if* you have SIBO with an antimicrobial (herbal) supplementation, real food and lifestyle change. If you respond positively to treatment, the likelihood of SIBO presence is indicated.

Intestinal Permeability (Leaky Gut)

Your intestinal barrier (surface and tissues) covers a surface area of 400 square meters and requires approximately 40 percent of the body's energy expenditure.

Your gut barrier helps keep nutrients housed in your digestive tract, prevents the loss of water (dehydration) and electrolytes, and inhibits the entry of "foreign invaders" (toxins, antigens, and microorganisms).

However, when your gut barrier is stressed, it impacts your health in multiple ways. Common diseases associated with "intestinal permeability" include:

- Gastric ulcers
- Diarrhea
- IBS & IBD
- Celiac disease and other autoimmune diseases
- Cancer (stomach, colon)
- Allergies
- Arthritis and inflammation
- Stubborn weight gain, obesity and metabolic dysfunction
- Neurological conditions (Parkinson's, Alzheimer's, etc.)
- Autism
- ADD/ADHD

There are many factors which affect the strength of your gut barrier system, including things like:

- Your nutrition (i.e. the Standard American Western diet, diet foods, lack of nutrients like proteins or healthy fats, or poor quality nutrients such as conventional meats and dairy)

- Lack of fermentable carbohydrates and fermented foods (probiotic and prebiotic foods); illnesses and toxins (bacterial, viral, parasitic infections, fungal overgrowth)
- Toxic exposure and overload (heavy metals, mycotoxins in bad coffee, mold)
- Medications (like PPI acid-suppressing drugs, birth control, antibiotics, statins, NSAIDs)
- Stressful lifestyle factors (like chronic stress, lack of sleep, too much or too little physical activity)

Intestinal permeability is almost always caused by something else (such as poor diet, gut infections, SIBO, bacterial overgrowth, chronic stress, etc.). If you do discover a "leaky gut," then by addressing these other factors in your protocol, leaky gut healing typically begins in conjunction.

For that reason, leaky gut testing is not always the first test I recommend.

Depending on symptoms, stool testing, SIBO, a comprehensive blood panel, and food intolerance testing can often give more detail as to what a triggering pathogen may be.

However, if other testing does not confirm positive results or if a gut healing protocol seems to be getting you nowhere, then an intestinal permeability screening can be a good assessment.

There are two primary methods of assessing leaky gut:

1. Lactulose-mannitol testing, and,
2. Antigenic permeability screen

The lactulose-mannitol test is a urine test involving measuring levels of these two sugars in the urine after the you take them orally. Since mannitol is small enough to pass directly through the cells, but lactulose is NOT small at all, the test evaluates if a healthy amount (10-30 percent) of mannitol is present in urine, and if less than 1 percent of lactulose is present. If results are abnormal, a leaky gut is suspected—mostly in the small intestine.

The antigenic permeability screen blood test is called Cyrex Array 2 through Cyrex Labs and evaluates the permeability of the entire length of the small intestine and large intestine. This screening triggers an autoimmune response in the body (body attacking itself) and assesses whether or not antibodies form. If they do, the likelihood of gut wall breakdown is common.

Of the two tests, due to the antigenic permeability screening giving a full-picture view of the digestive tract, it is my currently recommended test of choice.

Stool Test

Exactly what it sounds like: Assessing the bacterial cultures of your stool to see if there are any gut bugs that don't belong there (parasites, yeast, bacteria), identify root causes of GI symptoms, and assess for key markers of digestion, absorption, and inflammation.

While you will always have some gut bugs, you want more of the good guys than the bad guys hanging out. Parasites, foodborne disease organisms, and other fungal overgrowth bacteria can lie dormant in your GI tract for years beyond the food poisoning, parasite infection or stomach bug you caught as a kid, so the stool test helps identify those in order to kill them off.

The gold standard I recommend?

A high-complexity stool culture test such as the Doctor's Data Comprehensive Stool Test with Parasitology x 3 samples. In addition, BioHealth 401H is another reputable test to run alongside Doctor's Data to give you and your clinician a comprehensive evaluation of what gut bugs may be keeping your GI upset—with less room for error in test interpretations and results.

Together, the tests look at the bacterial composition of your gut flora, including any pathogens, dysbiotic species, or yeast that is present. In addition, it also helps assess your digestion, absorption, inflammation, and immune status; production of healthy amounts of short-chain fatty acids like butyrate and propionate; and the health of your blood and mucus.

If results come back positive, an antifungal, antimicrobial, or super-charged probiotic treatment protocol typically is prescribed—depending on your personal gut makeup.

Stool testing is an tremendously beneficial tool for making sure you are taking the **right probiotics for you.** Not all probiotics are beneficial—especially if you have an overgrowth of certain bacteria in your gut -- and stool testing can help you pick and choose supplements to help foster healthy bacteria (not overgrowth).

Candida Myth Buster

Candida is a bacterial yeast and is a NORMAL part of your GI tract—we all have it (just like we all have trillions of other bacteria as well).

Candida is not a bad thing, except when we have overgrowth of it—just like is the case with other bacteria.

Candida overgrowth and Candida cleanses became a popular diagnosis in the 1980s and 90s and has stuck around to this day.

To determine if you have Candida overgrowth, many nutritionists and holistic doctors will assess it based on if your tongue is white or your mucous in a cup of water does not sink to the bottom. If your tongue is white and/or the spit didn't sink, your practitioner may then confirm that you have Candida and prescribe you eat an anti-Candida (low carb) diet along with some antifungal supplements to kill the Candida.

Although some patients do report feeling better with such treatment, others report feeling worse, which begs the question: ***Are your gut symptoms really Candida overgrowth?***

Maybe not, for one of these three reasons:

1. Candida actually *can* also feed off of ketones (from low-carb diets)
2. When you're treating a bacterial overgrowth with antifungal supplements, you need to eat some real-food carbs (like sweet potatoes, fruits, etc.) to help bring the bacteria out to play—and be killed off
3. There may be MORE bacteria at play than just Candida

The Bottom Line: If you have bacterial overgrowth in your gut, it's important to know that Candida is NOT always the main bacteria to blame like once believed—and even if more Candida IS present, there may be hundreds of other bacteria at play as well. In this case, testing stool cultures and for SIBO are more likely to yield a more accurate assessment.

GI Scope

GI scope testing involves sending a camera into your GI tract to evaluate for structural damage, autoimmune disease (like Crohn's and Colitis), and cancer.

There are two types of "scopes" for assessing structural damage: Endoscopy (upper GI) and Colonoscopy (lower GI).

If you have an obstruction (blockage), structural damage, or some barrier preventing food from passing through your GI tract, in your large bowel or small intestine, a scope can pinpoint the problem. Common symptoms of GI blockage or structural damage of the GI tract are fairly similar to the symptoms you experience with other GI issues including bacterial overgrowth,

IBS, chronic indigestion, distension of the stomach depending on where the obstruction is located, abdominal pain and cramping, and more.

Who Should Do a Scope?
GI scopes, like colonoscopy testing, are highly invasive and is not recommended for testing and assessing your gut health state until other measures have been exhausted to address your underlying gut issues (the tests we've discussed and lifestyle factors).

Prior to your colonoscopy in particular, a 24 hour "prep diet" is prescribed, and includes clear liquids only and a high dose of over the counter laxatives to "clean you out." Common side effects from both the prep and procedure include bacterial dysbiosis and further gut imbalances.

Only if symptoms of GI health do not improve with other measures, is a GI scope highly recommended.

Ok…So what test should I run?!
Phew! That's a lot of different tests you can take.

Where to start?!

Before jumping into laboratory testing, I highly recommend you first establish a "baseline" with your 28-day gut kickstart. Let food and basic gut support essentials be thy medicine. After your 28 days, you'll have a clean slate and then may want to consider moving to labs if symptoms and gut issues persist.

EDIT: Additionally a SIBO test or experiment with a SIBO-healing protocol may be warranted, particularly if bloating after meals, malabsorption, loose stools/diarrhea, IBS, nutrient deficiencies, or constipation is present.

The primary tests I recommend most people start out with are:

1. Comprehensive Blood Chemistry
2. Comprehensive Stool Analysis

Additionally a SIBO test may be warranted, particularly if bloating after meals, malabsorption, loose stools/diarrhea, IBS, nutrient deficiencies, or constipation is present.

As for food intolerance testing, I typically first recommend 30 days of the Gut Kickstart protocol prior to any formal food intolerance testing to first self-test what foods you may be sensitive to. If you still can't determine which foods do and don't agree with you, then food intolerance testing may be warranted.

*** *Re-Test, Don't Guess!*
Ultimately, with testing (even your questionnaire), it's important to remember that re-assessment is a vital component to ensuring any changes or protocols are working, and is recommended 60-90 days after you've implemented any supplement, nutrition and lifestyle changes for healing. Many patients go through Part 1 (testing) and Part 2 (a prescribed gut-healing protocol) of the gut healing process, but fail to get a reassessment to see if their gut health improved.

Aye aye aye! I am overwhelmed!!!

Stop it right there! (and take a deep breath)…

Remember above all: Testing can help get to the deeper issues of your GI symptoms—(especially if you have been experiencing them for some time or you've "tried everything") BUT it does not trump the impact your lifestyle and LOVING YOUR GUT (from the inside out) can do for your own Gut Kickstart Protocol.

Phase 2: 28-Day Gut Kickstart

Assessments? Check.
Prepped? Check.
Jumpstart cleanse? Check.

After your Prep Week, you're ready to jump in to your 28 Day Gut Kickstart!

The Gut Kickstart is REALLY simple! There are really *only 3 essentials*-to focus on each week:

1. **Eat Real (Anti-inflammatory) Food**. Build your meals upon sustainable proteins, colorful veggies, and healthy fats that make your belly feel good. Minimize inflammatory foods. In addition, a few supplemental supports will help you get the most out of these foods.

2. **De-Stress.** If the gut is the gateway to health, then stress is the roadblock to health. You cannot supplement or eat your way out of a stressful lifestyle. Stress goes far beyond mental stress. It also includes physical stressors (like lack of sleep, overtraining or sedentary lifestyles, or too much screen exposure at night--sending your brain into hyperdrive mode). A stressed out body equals a stressed out gut, and for the next 28-Days you are going to focus on eliminating at least ONE stressor.

3. **Add in your 5 Daily "Gut Love Habits."** 5 essential habits for feeling good (inside and out) that will soon become second nature by the time your 28-Day Gut Kickstart is

said and done! You have 2 options for adding these to your daily routine: You can either start with ALL 5 Gut Love Habits from the beginning, or, if you're newer to gut healing, add ONE each week into your "Reintroduction" Phase. (See "Essential 3" in this chapter and "Resources" at the back of the book for a complete list of your habits).

Bonus: Boost Your Gut Health. Check out your Cheat Sheet Protocols in the Resources section at back of this book for additional supplemental support and protocols that can help you feel even better in your gut healing if you know you struggle with certain conditions (such as IBS, constipation, bloating, allergies or skin breakouts). These are completely optional and above all, your real food diet and 5 Daily Gut Love Habits will get you far.

Essential 1: Eat Real (Anti-inflammatory) Food

"Let food be thy medicine."—Hippocrates

Throughout your Gut Kickstart, you are going to do just that. No diets, crazy juice cleanses, bone-broth detoxes or restrictive mindsets included.

Eat *real* food—IN ABUNDANCE.

Foods your body was meant to thrive upon:

- Dark leafy greens
- Lots of fresh, colorful veggies
- Plant and animal fats
- Moderate sustainably raised meats and wild-caught fish
- Some colorful fruits
- No (added) sugar
- Lots of fresh, clean water

What is real food?!

Answer: If it didn't grow on the land, swim in the sea, or roam the earth, it's not real food.

These are the foods most often found on the outside edge of the grocery store, the Farmer's Market, or your great-great grandma's dinner plate. Simple foods your body was made to crave and digest (before Chic-Fil-A waffle fries confused your tastebuds and body).

Your Gut Kickstart is divided up into 3 different phases to help you figure out what foods work best for your body and digestion throughout the process—including your Pre-program Prep Week(s), 28-Day Reset, and bonus Reintroduction Phase. (Don't worry *too much* about the deets here. We'll cover em in Chapter 8).

Your 28-Day Gut Kickstart Nutrition Blueprint includes the following:

Gut Loving: 80%+ Foods (Eat Liberally)

- **Meat and Poultry.** Beef and lamb, but also chicken, turkey, duck and wild game like venison, ostrich, etc. Organic and free-range is always preferable. "Natural" means NOTHING.

- **Pastured Egg Yolks.**

- **Organ Meats (especially liver).** The most nutrient-dense food on the planet. If you don't like the taste of liver, one good trick is to put one chicken liver in each cube of an ice cube tray and freeze them. Then, when you're making any meat dish, dice up one chicken liver and add it to the meat.

- **Bone Broth & Meat Broth Soups.** Balance your intake of muscle meats and organ meats with homemade bone broths. Bone broths are rich in glycine and amino acid found in collagen, which is a protein important in maintaining a healthy gut lining.

- **Wild-Caught Fish.** Especially fatty fish like salmon, halibut, sardines, mackerel and herring. Wild is preferable. You need to eat three six-ounce servings of fatty fish per week to balance your omega-6 to omega-3 ratio.
- **Starchy Tubers.** Yams, sweet potatoes, yuca/manioc, winter squash, beets, carrots plantain, parsnips, etc.
- **Non-starchy Vegetables.** Cooked and raw. Especially dark leafy greens.
- **Fermented Vegetables and Fruits.** Sauerkraut, kimchi, beet kvass, coconut kefir, etc. These are excellent for gut health.
- **Fresh Fruit.** (1-2 servings/day). Especially berries and green-tipped bananas.
- **Traditional Fats.** Coconut oil, palm oil, lard, duck fat, beef tallow, and olive oil.
- **Prebiotic Veggies** (Roots & Starchy Tubers). Green tipped plantains, cooked & cooled potatoes/sweet potatoes, winter squash, jicama, garlic, onion, artichoke, roasted carrots, beets.
- **Olives, Avocados, & Coconut.** Including coconut milk- no additives, coconut butter, unsweetened coconut flakes.
- **Ghee & Grass-fed Butter.**
- **Sea Salt & Spices.**

*20%+ Not-Right-Now Foods (Eat Occasionally)**

- **Egg Whites.** Preferably pastured, free-range and/or organic. Why no eggs? Eggs are one of the top most allergenic foods. *Exception*: Pastured egg yolks which are less gut inflammatory.
- **Nuts & Seeds**. *Not* recommended for the first 28 days, as nuts are also more inflammatory foods. *Minimal small servings of sun-butter and seeds are easier to digest.* If you

do eat nuts, choose raw, soak overnight, then dehydrate or roast at low temperature (150 degrees) to improve digestibility. Favor nuts lower in omega-6, like hazelnuts and macadamias, and minimize nuts high in omega-6, like brazil nuts and almonds. No peanuts.

- **Pork.** The slowest digesting meat of all meats. Not suggested. If you do eat it, opt for pastured, organic sources.
- **Processed Meat, Sausage, Bacon & Jerky.** Make sure they are gluten, sugar, nitrate and soy-free; Organic/free-range meat is preferable.
- **Dried Fruit & Dates.** Depending on your blood sugar balance. These can be high in sugar. Opt for berries, bananas, citrus, pineapple, melons and other Low FODMAP fruits.
- **Nightshade Vegetables & Spices.** Tomatoes, white potatoes, eggplant, chili, peppers, cumin, paprika, red pepper flakes, etc.
- **Cruciferous & High FODMAP Veggies.** Brussels sprouts, broccoli, cauliflower, cabbage in limited quantities. Associated with more gas and bloating. Eat in limited amounts, or well-cooked and softened.
- **Coffee and Black Tea.** Black, or with coconut milk. Only if you don't suffer from fatigue, insomnia or hypoglycemia, and only before 12:00 PM. Limit to one cup/day (not one triple espresso - one cup).
- **Dark Chocolate.** 70 percent or higher in small amounts (i.e. about the size of a silver dollar per serving/day) is OK.
- **Restaurant Food.** The main problem with eating out is that restaurants often cook with industrial seed oils, which wreak havoc on the body and cause serious inflammation. You don't need to become a cave dweller, but it's best to limit eating out as much as possible during this initial period.

- **Dairy.** Keep dairy foods, like cheese, conventional yogurt, milk, cream and any dairy product which comes from a cow, goat or sheep to a minimum to distill any inflammation. *Exception*: Grass-fed butter, ghee and grass-fed yogurt/Goat's Milk yogurt as tolerated (since much of the lactose is extracted); Opt for coconut yogurt, additive-free unsweetened coconut milk or almond milk.
- **Grains.** Including bread, rice, cereal, oats, pasta or any "gluten-free" pseudo grains like sorghum, teff, quinoa, amaranth, buckwheat, etc. *Exception:* Cooked & cooled Jasmine white rice; Grain substitues: coconut flour, almond flour, tapioca starch.
- **Legumes.** Including beans of all kinds (soy, black, kidney, pinto, etc.), peas, lentils and peanuts. *Exception*: Green Peas, Sugar Snap Peas.
- **Natural Sweeteners.** Minimal raw honey and pure maple syrup, Minimal true green leaf stevia
- **Gluten-Free Processed Foods.** The only thing missing? Gluten. Many of these products are still as processed.
- **"Paleo-Friendly" Packaged Foods & Baked Goods.** Healthy, yes. But, same as the gluten-free processed foods…still in moderation. Build you plate first on sustainable proteins, greens and healthy fats—then adding in the occasional coconut flour tortillas,

Gut Inflammatory Foods (Not Advised!)

The following foods are recommended to keep to a <u>***minimum (if at all)***</u>. No, you cannot live in a bubble, but mindfulness with the fuel you put in to your body will directly impact your brain, gut, and energy health!

- **Processed or Refined Foods.** As a general rule, if it comes in a bag or a box, don't eat it. This also includes highly processed "health foods" like protein powder, energy bars, dairy-free creamers, etc.

- **Sugar & Artificial Sweeteners.** Including sugar, high-fructose corn syrup, agave, brown rice syrup, Splenda, Equal, Nutrasweet.
- **Industrial Seed Oils.** Soybean, corn, safflower, sunflower, cottonseed, canola, etc. Read labels - seed oils are in almost all processed, packaged and refined foods (which you should be mostly avoiding anyway).
- **Sodas & Diet Sodas.** All forms.
- **Alcohol**. In any form. (Don't freak out. It's just 30 days.)
- **Processed Sauces & Seasonings**. Soy sauce, tamari, and other processed seasonings and sauces (which often have sugar, soy, gluten, or all of the above).

Why These Specific Food Recommendations?!

The foods listed in the 80% category of your Gut Love Nutrition Blueprint are anti-inflammatory foods. However this doesn't mean the list of 20% foods are unhealthy for you.

Instead, these recommendations are meant to help you recognize what is (or isn't) be healthy for your body right NOW in terms of gut health.

For example, foods like nuts, eggs and broccoli are very healthy foods, but if you have an underlying gut issue, they may be more inflammatory to your gut due to lectins and phytates (nuts), lysozyme and albumin (enzyme and protein in egg whites that trigger leaky gut), or fructan sugars (FODMAP foods like broccoli).

You don't have to eat McDonald's Big Macs or Doritos chips for digestive issues to arise. Every body is different, and if you have an underlying or unaddressed gut issue or imbalance, certain foods (even healthy foods) may not sit with your gut.

If you ever struggle with wondering WHY healthy eating hurts, this may help.

Here are 10 foods which can be hard to digest (even though they are "healthy"):

1. Green Juice & Smoothies
Green juice and smoothies are packed with nutrients! However, due to their rapidly digesting nature, as well as temperature (often served cold), they can prove difficult for some to digest. In addition, sometimes smoothies are often packed with lots of fruit, which can be a big shot of rapidly digesting fructose (sugar) in one setting. Additionally, when fruit is combined with other more complex, slow digesting foods—like proteins or fats—the gut and liver wage war on your digestive tract to work with two speeds at once (fast digesting fruit and slow digesting proteins and fats). Sugar in fruit also sticks to proteins--too much of either at once leads to a "sticky" situation. As for other ingredients—it may be an ingredient or two itself that just does not sit with you (like almond butter or almond milk—especially with additives, a can of full fat coconut milk or certain veggies—such as kale, celery, or beets.

Gut Hack: Play around with combos of smoothies and keep them simple. If you've been using the same base (and not always feeling well)—like coconut milk, almond milk, coconut water, milk, etc.—try a different kind of milk (avoid soy and conventional dairy as they are well known gut irritants). Throw in a green of choice—like spinach, and try your smoothie with fruit and without fruit. Mix up your protein powders (hemp, additive-free beef isolate, collagen) and different types of add-ins (cinnamon, cocoa, lemon, ginger, etc.) and fats (avocado, coconut oil, MCT oil, nutbutters). Do something different until you find a good combo for you. While you're at it, throw in some probiotics (the powder from one of your capsules or some kefir or low-sugar kombucha) and try sipping slowly over the course of 15-30 minutes (as opposed to 5-minutes) or drinking half what you usually drink.

2. Nuts & Nut Butters
"Nut gut" happens when you take a good thing a little overboard—at least for your digestive system's tolerance. Common side effects of poor nut digestion include: Frequent constipation, gas, stomach cramping, bloating, skin breakouts, environmental allergies, low immunity, unexplained or "stubborn" weight gain, a "slow metabolism," and insatiable cravings for nuts and nutbutters (despite not feeling well). While too many nuts can irritate the gut lining, you are more susceptible to the impacts of "nut gut" if there was already an underlying digestive imbalance in the first place.

Why does nut gut happen? Like grains, most nuts also contain indigestible compounds—phytates and lectins—meant to protect a nut in the wild from predators and weather. Hence, when we eat nuts, we consume this "armor" on the outer shell of the nut, and our body has a hard time breaking it down. The phytic acid composition (from phytates) in nuts also prevents the absorption of vitamins and minerals found in nuts in the first place. It is often called an "anti-nutrient"—as if you eat the nut, but you get zero benefit from it because it is indigestible to your body.

Gut Hack: Soak nuts overnight and dry or roast them before consuming (it can promote better digestion) to see if that makes a difference; Or consider taking a break from nuts to address underlying gut imbalances then come back and see if it helps.

Nut-Free Snack Ideas
- Kale chips with extra virgin olive or "Kale Krunch"
- Rainbow carrot "fries" + homemade paleo aioli
- Cucumbers + guacamole
- Parsnip "fries" with olive oil or duck fat
- Plantain chips with guacamole or organic salami
- Jicama slices with coconut yogurt
- Green apple or pear slices with coconut butter
- Cauliflower "popcorn" (homemade)
- Homemade zucchini "chips" with paleo ranch dressing
- Celery with sunbutter
- Roasted beet "chips"
- Roasted sweet potato "chips" (or Jackson's Honest chips) with homemade Tzatziki sauce or paleo honey mustard
- Kelp chips and seaweed snacks
- Tigernuts
- Homemade apple "chips" with cinnamon and coconut oil
- Toasted coconut chips
- Seeds (pumpkin, sunflower)
- Coconut flour tortilla chips with guacamole
- Roasted veggies drizzled with avocado oil
- Turkey or grass-fed beef jerky

3. Salad

Raw leafy greens play a leading role in your 28-Day Gut Kickstart protocol—except when you can't digest them well. Unlike cooked leafy greens, raw leafy greens take an extra step to digest if you don't have the proper enzymes to break them down. Some veggies (like raw leafy greens) are high in *insoluble* fiber. While soluble fiber can be soothing for the gut, when we eat larger amounts of insoluble fiber (especially if our gut is already inflamed) it is like rubbing a brush on an open wound. It hurts our gut. Other veggies that may fall into this category include: Green beans, bell peppers, eggplant, celery, onions, broccoli, Brussels sprouts, broccoli, and cauliflower.

Gut Hack: Try mixing up your consumption of raw and cooked leafy greens—sometimes have raw, sometimes have cooked. Warm salads are still delicious (or pre-cooked greens that you let cool). Saute greens in coconut oil or ghee to soften with a touch of sea salt, then place in fridge if you want it cooler prior to consumption. In addition, consider adding a little soluble fiber to your salads to also make them more digestible (like butternut squash, sweet potatoes, beets, roasted carrots, etc.), as well as a fermented food (sauerkraut, fermented veggies). Remove the stems from foods like broccoli and cauliflower.

4. Apples

An apple a day keeps the doctor away—except when you feel like the whole apple (or watermelon or pear or banana) is sitting in your gut. If you're prone to bloating, some fruits (especially FODMAP foods and fruits) can trigger gut symptoms. FODMAP is an acronym that stands for Fermentable Oligosaccharides, Disaccharides, Monosaccharides And

Polyols. In short: FODMAPS are foods which are indigestible short-chain carbohydrates, or sugar molecule. Since your body is unable to completely digest these sugar molecules, they travel through your GI tract and reach your colon undigested, where the bacteria that live in your colon begin to ferment them. If you have bacteria overgrowth in particular, the fermentation can produce gas and bloating. Other common FODMAP foods include: Onions, cruciferous veggies (broccoli, cauliflower, brussels sprouts), garlic, sugar alcohols (xylitol, mannitol and sorbitol), beans/legumes (including peanuts), dairy, and grains.

Gut Hack: Try Low-FODMAP fruits to see if that makes a difference. Also consider consuming fruit alone since the sugars in fruit digest faster than other foods you eat.

Low-FODMAP Fruits
Banana
Blueberries
Grapefruit
Kiwi
Lemon
Lime
Mandarin
Melons (including cantaloupe and honeydew)
Orange
Papaya
Passionfruit
Pineapple
Raspberries
Rhubarb
Strawberries

5. Eggs

Like "nut gut," egg belly is real. Eggs are one of the top eight 'most allergenic' foods—along with milk, nuts, peanuts, and soy (all of which account for 90% of all food reactions). Even if you don't have a diagnosed allergy by an allergist, there is a reason eggs don't always sit well with folks (particularly if you are already susceptible to a leaky gut): Upon digestion, the albumin protein in the egg white can often slip past the intestinal wall and get in your body and can cause a reaction. Additionally, lysozyme is a proteolytic enzyme in egg whites that can be challenging on the gut as they may lead to increased permeability.

Common reactions or signs of egg intolerance include runny sinuses, brain fog, cramping, bloating and/or diarrhea. Folks who are sensitive to eggs are also often sensitive to several other 'inflammatory' foods, like nuts, grains, dairy, and gluten.

Gut Hack: Remove eggs from your diet for 21-30 days while implementing your Gut Kickstart digestive protocol then reintroduce. See how you feel. Try duck eggs. Eat just the yolks—see how you feel. Try homemade turkey or chicken sausage, salmon or leftovers from dinner for breakfast instead.

6. Coconut

Coconut is often a staple fat source for many who have turned to a real food diet. However, unfortunately for some, coconut is a FODMAP food which can trigger similar reactions as some experience with apples due to fructose malabsorption (bloating, gas, pain, constipation or diarrhea). This results in enhanced levels of undigested fructose in your gut, which then causes the overgrowth of bacteria in your small intestine. Undigested fructose also reduces the absorption of water into the intestine. Additionally, some forms of coconut milk contain more than just the coconut—sugars, additives and BPA's from the cans, for instance. Look for additive-free and BPA-free coconut milk with just coconut, water, possibly guar gum as an experiment.

Gut Hacks: Try different forms of coconut and see if you feel differently (coconut milk vs. light coconut milk, coconut butter, coconut oil, etc.). Replace coconut oil and coconut butter with ghee, nut butter or grass-fed butter. Drizzle extra virgin olive oil on veggies or salads. Try coconut kefir or goat's milk kefir instead of coconut milk. Dilute coconut water or coconut milk with water.

7. Beets

Beets are highly touted in the gut-healing world as being super detoxifying for your liver and digestive system. Beets contain a few gut-supportive components including betaine (which helps your liver cells eliminate toxins), pectin (a fiber which clears toxins that have been removed from the liver so they don't re-invade the body), and betalains (pigments with high anti-inflammatory properties to encourage the detoxification process). However, too much of a good thing at once can be a "not-so-good thing"—especially if your liver is congested or not ready to fully "cleanse" yet (due to other gut issues). Beets are a very healthy food, but are best incorporated into your diet in small doses to build up your gut and liver tolerance for digesting them. In addition, if your body is low in stomach acid, you may notice red or pink-colored urine when you eat beets since beets contain betalain pigments. If stomach acid is low, you can't break down these pigments as easily (although you may not experience digestive symptoms).

Gut Hack: Introduce beets in medicinal amounts every other day or few days over the course of a week or two. Drink 4-6 ounces of beet juice as opposed to 10-16 ounces in a smoothie. Support your liver health, stomach acid and digestive system by incorporating fermented foods, probiotics/prebiotics, digestive enzymes and addressing any bacterial overgrowth with antimicrobial.

8. Bone Broth

Bone broth is considered a "gut healing" food due to its rich amino acid and gelatin/collagen profile. However, if you have a leaky gut or poor gut health already, bone broth can sometimes be too strong of a gut healer, since it is also a "high histamine" food. Bone broth—directly from bones of chicken, beef or fish—contains a power-punch of nutrients as well as histamine —a neurotransmitter which plays an important role in keeping your immune system, digestion, and nervous system working right. For most people, the amount of histamine in a food simply isn't an issue, and if your system is working right, it immediately inactivates any histamine you don't need. But if you have a chronic leaky gut and are intolerant to histamine, then foods like bone broth are an overkill to your gut and your body is UNABLE to get rid of any histamine you don't need (firing up symptoms even more—like bloating, brain fog, gas or constipation). Additionally, the quality of the bones and length of time you cook them make a difference. It's no secret organic, pastured and grass-fed meats contain more nutrients than conventional bones and we eat what our animals eat (toxins included). Also, over cooking your bones or long cooking times of bone broth is not good for some. Bone broth typically simmers at a low temperature for many hours, long enough to allow the connective tissues to dissolve and the minerals to be drawn into the broth. Chicken bone broth needs to cook 6 to 24 hours. Beef broth needs at least 24-72 hours to ensure all the cartilage and tendons dissolve. (The bigger the bone, the longer it takes.) The result of such long cooking times is a tremendous amount of glutamic acid. If you already have a leaky gut, too much of this acid is linked to brain fog, bloating, constipation, loose stools and feeling less than stellar.

Gut Hack: Make sure your bone broth is made with real (organic) meat bones. Add some healthy fat to your bone broth—like grass-fed butter or ghee—to aid in digestion. Try meat broth instead—the whole chicken cooked in the crockpot (has lower in histamine and glutamic acid).

9. Sauerkraut

Fermented foods, like sauerkraut, are natural probiotics said to be rich in "healthy probiotics." However, since sauerkraut is a fermented food, if you do have bacterial overgrowth in your gut, bacteria love feasting on fermented foods (i.e. yeast). If you're not supporting your gut with a supplemental approach to help kill off bacterial overgrowth, then cramping, bloating, diarrhea or constipation could be a side effect of your bacteria's Thanksgiving meal. It's also important to note that it may not be the sauerkraut itself, but your simple lack of digestion of that sauerkraut because you don't have prebiotics to go with it! Prebiotics are what "feed" your probiotics in order to stick in your gut and can be found in some foods, as well as in supplemental form.

Gut Hack: Test, don't guess. If fermented foods make you feel bloated or gassy, test to see if you have SIBO (small intestinal bacterial overgrowth), or an imbalance on an Organic

Acids Test (D-Lactate levels will often be "off" in response to lactic acid bacteria), hinting at SIBO, gut infection or "leaky gut." Take a break from fermented foods and stick to your soil-based probiotics, along with digestive enzymes during meals.

10. Cassava Flour
Gas, constipation and bloating are common side effects from cassava or tapioca starch, which is commonly used in baked goods and gluten-free goods (even "paleo" friendly). Tapioca is a cross-reactive food with gluten, containing many similar proteins found in gluten-containing grains and can cause backup to happen if your gut can't break it down.

Gut Hack: Use a different real-food flour that does not cross-contaminate with gluten (like coconut flour or arrowroot starch) and make sandwiches on lettuce wraps or coconut flour tortillas. Instead of baked goods, wraps and breads, focus on eating mostly real foods (veggies and starchy veggies, and some fruits) during your 28-Day Gut Kickstart for your carbohydrate sources.

The Bottom Line:
How does your body feel?

Whatever you eat may be totally "healthy" according to health standards, but if there is an underlying imbalance, it may not be the food for you—right now.

In addition, often times the stress we feel about eating alone can cause digestive upset. If you are worried or stressed that a certain food is going to make you feel badly, what do you think will happen? When you approach meals with an open mindedness, breath, and a posture of acceptance (accepting nourishing food), you may very well surprise yourself what happens.

The bottom line: Address any underlying gut imbalances (along with stress), and you may feel better when you reintroduce these foods.

The 28 Day Gut Kickstart Meal Template

Here's what three meals per day may consist of:

Water Intake: Clean, filtered water or mineral water: half of your bodyweight in ounces throughout the day

Pre-Breakfast
16 oz. warm water (optional: lemon + sea salt)
1 tbsp. Apple Cider Vinegar in 2-4 oz. water (add pinch of raw honey if this is completely unbearable)

Breakfast
Choose one of the following two options:
Protein: 4-6 oz.
Fat: 1-2 servings
Vegetables (Consume leafy greens at least 2x per day, cooked, in a smoothie, or raw)
Recommended Gut Love Habits:
    Digestive Enzymes: 1-2
or

Morning Sips (if not a breakfast person):
- Butter Bones + Collagen + Ghee

- Smoothie: Lite Coconut Milk or Water + Greens + 1 Scoop Beef Isolate or Collagen with Carob Powder + 1/2 Green-tipped Banana or Berries + 1/3 Avocado
- Coconut or Goat's Milk Yogurt + Fruit "Parfait" (Fruit of Choice + Tiger Nuts or Toasted Coconut Chips + Cinnamon + 1/4 tsp. pure Vanilla)
- Golden Tea: Ginger turmeric tea blended with Coconut Milk or Ghee + Scoop Collagen + Drizzle pure maple syrup (optional)

Lunch
Protein: 4-6 oz.
Fat: 1-2 servings
Vegetables
Recommended Gut Love Habits:
   Digestive Enzymes: 1-2 (optional)
   1 Tbsp. Apple Cider Vinegar in 2-4 oz. water (optional)

Dinner—aim to eat at least 2-3 hours before bed
Protein: 4-6 oz.
Fat: 1-2 servings
Vegetables
Recommended Gut Love Habits:
   Digestive Enzymes: 1-2 (optional)
   1 Tbsp. Apple Cider Vinegar in 2-4 oz. water (optional)

Bed-time
8 oz. Herbal Tea (ginger, peppermint or licorice root)

Snack (Optional: Mid-Morning or Afternoon)

Only snack if your energy needs and hunger-fullness demand it. The point of the Gut Kickstart Program is NOT to go hungry, but to balance your blood sugar and brain-gut connection (connected with your true hunger-and-fullness cues). Three balanced meals per day allows your body adequate time to digest your foods. Snacking is not a bad thing, but chances are, if you focus on eating balanced meals—with enough protein, fat and veggies in them—you may find you don't need snacks like you once did and you are plenty satisfied. See Snack Ideas in your Resources.

Gut Love Meal Protocol Notes

Fermented Foods. Incorporate 1-2 fermented foods in condiment-sized servings each day in your daily diet. These may include sauerkraut, fermented veggies, kimchi, fermented yogurt or kefir, and kvass.

Fruits & Starches: Aim for 2-3 different colors in each meal between veggies, starchy veggies and occasional fruit. You may incorporate 1-2 fruits per day and 1-2 starchy vegetables (like sweet potatoes or squashes) where you see fit. Starchy veggies and tubers contain essential prebiotic fibers for helping you be more "regular." Fruit is typically best digested when eaten alone or paired with easy-to-digest foods like a smoothie, yogurt or light salad. Easier-to-digest fruits include green-tipped bananas, cooked or softened apples and pears, and berries.

Water: Continue to drink water throughout the day, aiming for half your bodyweight in ounces of clean, filtered water. La Croix, Topo Chico, juice, Crystal Light or any other beverage do not count as water. You may add citrus, lemon, cucumber, mint, berries or any other fruit you like to your water if you like.

Vegetables: Consume leafy greens with at least two meals, along with other non-starchy vegetables if you like. Cooked veggies often digest better than raw, so keep that in mind. Keep starchy veggies to approximately 1-2 servings per day, such as a sweet potato with some cooked greens at dinner, or a butternut squash hash with ground turkey and kale at breakfast. (If you are more active, training 4-6 days per week, then two starches per day is recommended).

Sample Meal Day During Your 28-Day Gut Kickstart:

Pre-Breakfast
16 oz. warm water (optional: lemon + sea salt)
1 tbsp. Apple Cider Vinegar in 2-4 oz. water (add pinch of raw honey if this is completely unbearable)

Breakfast
Turkey Sausage
1/2 Avocado
Pan-fried Greens in 1 tbsp. of Ghee

Lunch
Canned Wild-Salmon
Leafy Greens
Roasted Beets
2 Tbsp. Coconut Butter
Oil & Vinegar Dressing
Sauerkraut

Snack (Optional)
8 oz. of Bone Broth

Dinner—aim to eat at least 2-3 hours before bed
Herb Crusted Chicken Thighs (skin on)
Sauteed Spinach in 1 tbsp. of ghee
Roasted Rainbow Carrots
Sauerkraut or other Fermented Vegetable (medicinal serving, 2-3 forkfuls)

Bedtime
8 oz. Herbal Tea
Goat's Milk or Coconut Kefir + Blueberries

*See your the Gut Kickstart Resources section at the back of the book for meal ideas and a comprehensive list of foods to eat in abundance.

How Much Should I Eat?: Portion Sizes
If you are eating liberal and adequate portions at meals, you may find you feel fueled longer throughout the day. Here are general portion size recommendations—no measuring needed!

- Protein:1-2 palm sizes
- Veggies: Half your plate
- Fat: 1/2 avocado, 1-2 spoonfuls (tablespoons) of oils and nut butters, handful of nuts
- Starches (potatoes, winter squash, carrots): Size of your fist
- Fruit: Size of your fist
- Fermented Foods: ¼ cup - ½ cup serving

Food Quality Matters
On top of eating real food, food quality matters. You wouldn't put cheap gas in a Ferrari, would you? Well your body is a Ferrari. To ensure top quality goes into your tank, opt for quality sources that make your body feel good.

- Reach for real organic, grass-fed, pasture-raised and wild-caught real foods (not necessarily "organic Oreos" and "organic Mac & Cheese").
- Eat 17-18 home cooked meals (80%) per week. Many restaurants cook their food in vegetable oils (hydrogenated oils, margarine) which clog up your gut like Crisco

in your kitchen sink, and sneak in sugars in unexpected places—like sauces and salad dressings.
- If eaten, soak nuts, grains and seeds in water prior to consumption.
- Wash veggies and fruits thoroughly before consuming.
- Food lasts about three days once prepared (in the fridge). Freeze leftovers if you need to.

Basic Gut Love: Supplements

During your first 28 days, we are taking a "minimalist" approach—aiming to get the majority of your gut support from food itself with a few additional supplement boosters. (These are actually included into your 5 Daily Gut Love Habits as well). Here's your list:

Supplement List

1. Soil Based Probiotic
2. Prebiotic Fiber (like Partially Hydrolyzed Guar Gum)
3. Digestive Enzymes (use as needed)
4. Gut Healing Foods:
    - Apple Cider Vinegar or HCL Tablet (if not pregnant or taking PPIs)
    - Fermented & Prebiotic Foods (as tolerated)

Here's how to take them:

Pre-Breakfast
12-16 oz. warm lemon water
1 Probiotic

Breakfast
1-2 Digestive Enzymes
Apple Cider Vinegar (1 tbsp in water) or HCL Tablet with Betaine & Pepsin (600-700 mg)

Lunch
1-2 Digestive Enzymes
Apple Cider Vinegar (1 tbsp in water) or HCL Tablet with Betaine & Pepsin (600-700 mg)

Dinner
1-2 Digestive Enzymes
Apple Cider Vinegar (1 tbsp in water) or HCL Tablet with Betaine & Pepsin (600-700 mg)

Before Bed
Prebiotic 1-2 tsp in 8 oz water or tea
Probiotic
Herbal Tea

Consume 1-2 condiment sized servings of a probiotic food and prebiotic food each day

PROBIOTIC FERMENTED FOODS

*eat in medicinal servings (2-3 forkfuls)

- Sauerkraut
- Fermented Veggies (carrots, beets, cucumber relish, dill pickles, etc.)
- Pickled Veggies (no added sugar or additives)
- Fermented Salsa
- Fermented Horseradish
- Goat's Milk Yogurt & Kefir
- Coconut Kefir
- Water Kefir
- Coconut Yogurt (no additives)
- Low-Sugar Kombucha (2-3 grams per serving)
- Beet Kvass
- Kimchi

PREBIOTIC FOODS

- Apple Cider Vinegar
- Asparagus (al dente)
- Banana (Green-tipped)
- Cooked & Cooled Jasmine white rice
- Cooked & Cooled Parsnips, Winter Squash, Carrots
- Cooked & Cooled Sweet Potatoes/Potatoes
- Dandelion greens
- Eggplant
- Endive
- Fennel
- Garlic
- Raw Honey
- Jerusalem artichokes
- Jicama
- Kefir
- Leeks
- Legumes
- Onions
- Peas
- Plantains (green-tipped)
- Radicchio
- Mushrooms (reishi, shiitake and maitake)
- Nutritional Yeast
- Potato Starch or Plantain Starch
- Seaweed/Algae

Q. Is this forever?! I'm not sure I can eat "clean" forever…
What is possible in 28 days? Dare yourself to find out.

Your initial Gut Kickstart Nutrition Blueprint is intended for your 28-Day Gut Kickstart. At the end of your 28 days, you will be guided in how to begin reintroducing foods from the other lists and being a sleuth (with yourself) to see what foods do (or do not) impact your overall gut wellness. Above all, keep in mind that 80/20 balance is essential!

80/20 Balance 101
While this list may seem "impossible" or strict for some, keep in mind: You have TOTAL permission to NOT be perfect!

Unlike most other diets, cleanses, or protocols out there that focus solely on what you "should" and "shouldn't" eat, the 28-Day Gut Kickstart challenges you to STOP being so hard on yourself when it comes to healing or changing your body. Instead, reconnect to the natural born language you've known all along: your gut intuition.

Remember: Stress or war with our bodies and food can only perpetuate the distress in our body and gut. No wonder more than 95 percent of diets—even "healthy eating" diets, like AIP, GAPS, SCD and more—fail over time!

(P.S.: Did you know the word "diet" actually means "a way of life?")

The ultimate aim of the Gut Kickstart is to help you (and your gut) find a "way of life" which is both nourishing and feels good—inside and out.

During the protocol, your goal is to **eat REAL FOOD the _majority_ of the time—at least 80%.** The other **20% of the time? Let life happen**.

- When in Rome, try the pasta.
- Out to eat? Do the best you can—even if organic is unavailable.
- Running out the door and forgot breakfast? Get something healthy on the go.

The 20 percent foods are called "not right now" foods because they are more highly associated with gut inflammation. Do your best to minimize these foods, (so you can have a REALLY ACCURATE idea of if your body tolerates them or not during your post-28 day "reintroduction" phase), but at the same time, feel free.

I challenge you to continually ask yourself throughout your program: *"How do I feel?"*

I call this the "Gut Check Method."

The Gut Check Method

Like a sixth sense, the **Gut Check Method** *involves honing the skill and ability to tune in with yourself anytime you feel overwhelmed, stressed, sad, anxious, constipated, bloated, crampy, hungry, frustrated, or confused (about what to eat, what to do, etc.).*

It's about listening to your gut—and training yourself to naturally do that again if you've lost that skill.

Listening to your gut is a skill you were born with—something deep within you.

You and your body are wired not just to survive, but to thrive, and as a baby, you totally knew how to listen to yourself and your body to do just that.

- *You cried when your gut was hungry, sad or upset.*
- *You laughed when you were tickled.*
- *You fussed when your gut was unhappy, gassy, bubbly or no one was listening to you.*
- *You felt content when your body was nourished—butt wiped clean and you slept well.*

- *You cooed when your mom or dad showed you affection and felt confidently loved through their touch and care for your needs.*

*You were totally in check with your **gut—in more ways than one**.*

*"Listening to your gut," (and healing your gut) also goes far beyond the digestive tract, supplements or lab tests. The "Gut Check Method" involves listening to your body, your mind **and** your heart.*

These three parts are all connected and when we tap into the power of our mind and our heart as part of our gut-healing, paired with our physical body healing, we take our healing to another level.

For instance, checking in with your gut feelings (heart), may look like:

- *Saying "no" sometimes instead of saying "yes" all the time—and saving yourself lots of stress in the long run.*
- *Going after your passions and goals—instead of passively thinking about them or hating your job.*
- *Acknowledging your loneliness in isolation and seeking to build and strengthen your friendships.*
- *Not trying to be all things to all people, but instead focusing on being the best you.*
- *Reflecting if your current lifestyle is aligning with what it is you really want.*
- *Assessing whether the need for coffee or chocolate is a craving or healthy dose.*
- *Quieting the worry running rampant in your mind with the words, "worry is negative imagination."*
- *Believing and seeing your own opportunity for healing and GI relief.*

***FUN FACT:** 90 percent of your serotonin "feel good" brain chemicals are produced in your gut. When our guts feel good—or better—our brains feel better, and vice versa!*

Gut Checking *also involves seeing yourself where you want to be, or imagining who healthy, thriving, vibrant, symptom-free you is. What does he or she...*

- *Feel like?*
- *Act like?*
- *Treat his body like?*
- *Eat? Not eat?*
- *Speak like (to himself)?*
- *How does she listen to herself?*
- *Is she optimistic or pessimistic?*

Get a clear picture of who healthy, thriving, gut-symptoms-free you is and pretend to be him or her.

You are your (and your gut's) best advocate.

As you embody her in your heart and head, you will become her (sans bloating or constipation) and you may find that your symptoms subside.

So as we think, therefore we become.

The placebo effect is for real, and psychological interventions (like positive thinking, self-talk, and hypnosis) alone have been shown to treat and remediate severe gut issues like IBS and inflammatory bowel diseases (Ballou & Keefer, 2017) even more than conventional medical treatments.

*Plus, you **already** know (deep down in your gut) what it is that feels right, doesn't feel right, sits right, and doesn't sit right.*

- *You know what foods digest well and what foods do not.*

- *You know when overwhelm or stress carries you away and what recenters you.*
- *You know when you feel better and when you feel worse.*
- *You know when your gut is telling you to do something (chase your passion) or not do something (turn down the opportunity).*
- *You know when it's a craving you can handle or a craving that will lead to a binge*
- *You know if your supplement routine is helping our not.*
- *You know when you keep saying "yes" to everything, you get burned out and that you need boundaries.*
- *You know when you're hungry or if you're just eating because you're bored.*

The problem is…we forget to check in. We forget to use this most powerful skill we've known all of our lives and we're not connected. Until now.

You ALREADY have the key to unlocking your "gut issues" when you get connected to your gut (heart, head and body).

You've simply forgotten what it means to check-in (and listen) to that gut. Until now.

Implementing the Gut Check Method
The Gut Check Method Involves three simple steps:

Step 1: Halt. Stop the thoughts. Slow down.
Step 2: Breathe. Take 5 deep breaths—in through your nose and out through your mouth. Relax your forehead, your worry, your stressed out brain or gut.
Step 3: Dig deep. Close your eyes. And check in: What do I need or want?

That's it. Anytime overwhelm, confusion or complicated protocols or questions tempt to thwart you—check in and get back to

> *keeping it simple (and simple answers). Don't worry, you'll get lots of practice with this skill!*

Clean Water

Water is the MOST important nutrient for human life. You can survive several weeks without food, but your body can only go approximately seven days without water. Your body alone is comprised of 60 percent or more of water, so in order for all the bodily processes inside you to function optimally, **you need to water your body (like a plant needs water) for processes such as:**

- Viscosity and healthy blood flow
- Healthy digestion
- Easing constipation
- Elimination of waste
- Assimilation and delivery of nutrients
- Brain power, focus and function
- Regulated appetite
- Energy
- Warding off sickness

The baseline amount for water intake is **half your bodyweight in ounces of water.** And not just any water, but **clean, pure (filtered) drinking water.**

Although water purification plants take steps to *minimize* toxins, more than 1,100 toxic compounds have been identified in our daily drinking water across the U.S.—including pesticides and metals like lead and mercury. These toxins are linked to varying chronic and debilitating diseases, such as: Alzheimer's, asthma, most forms of cancer, infertility, Parkinson's and arthritis.

The best source?

The gold standard is purified drinking water through filtration systems that help remove extra filth, dirt and toxins from our water. Technically speaking, anything called a "purifier" by industry standards must remove 99.75 percent of incoming bacteria (a pretty steep requirement). You can easily buy a water filter for your faucet, filtered water bottle, or an entire filtration system for your household.

Other notable water mentions (in order of best to least favored), include:
- Spring Water
- Mineral Water
- *Some* bottled waters. **Note:** Don't be fooled thinking the bottled water in your local supermarket are all "safe" for you. Many companies have actually been caught bottling tap water (See the Environmental Working Group's Bottled Water Scorecard on their website www.ewg.com)
- Well Water
- And the worst: Unfiltered Tap Water.

While COMPLETELY avoiding toxic exposure in our water is impossible, by choosing to arm your drinking, bathing and cleaning water supply with a filtration system, you are two (hundred) steps ahead.

Focus 2: De-Stress

Stress wreaks havoc on our health (both physical and mental stressors). Consider what stressors are present in your life, and at least one that you'd want to tackle the next 28-Days by cutting it out, or bringing it back to balance.

Physical Stressors

- Bluelight screen exposure (long times on screens)
- Light at night time
- Less than 7 hours of sleep most nights
- Overtraining
- Sedentary lifestyle
- Imbalanced exercise (i.e. doing HIIT or chronic cardio all the time without mixing it up)
- Exposure to chemicals in beauty, cleaning and hygiene products
- Plastic Tupperware/container use and other environmental toxins
- Mold exposure
- Lack of outdoor/nature and fresh air
- Endlessly Google searching answers to your health questions
- NSAID use (headaches, etc.)
- Oral birthcontrol and/or long term prescription medication use
- Disconnection from community/meaningful relationships
- High coffee/caffeine consumption (more than 1 cup quality coffee/day)
- Disrupted circadian rhythms for sleeping, eating, working and resting patterns
- Artificial sweeteners (most commercial stevia included)
- Eating packaged, refined or processed foods
- Low water intake (less than half your bodyweight in ounces)
- Tap water (not filtered)
- High alcohol consumption or smoking
- Frequent eating out (more than preparing/handling your food)

- Stress over food/diet
- Under-eating
- Low fiber (Fermentable prebiotic fiber foods)
- Lack of quality protein (amino acids for your brain)
- Conventional meat and dairy consumption
- Grains and "gluten free" processed products (with gluten-cross contaminants)
- Binging/Purging and disordered eating habits
- Jet lag
- Shift work
- Pain (joint, musculoskeletal)
- Infectious/bacterial disease
- Gut inflammation & Underlying gut conditions (SIBO, parasites, etc.)

Mental Stressors

- Type A personality—and difficulty listening to your body over your schedule
- Relationship stress
- Financial stress/
- Lack of control
- Burnout
- Not talking about your stress (bottling it up)
- Lack of play/fun
- Not doing things you love
- Serotonin suppression ("feel good" brain chemicals)
- Social Media comparison/endless scrolling
- Trying to be all things to all people/people pleasing
- FOMO (lack of downtime for yourself)
- Burning a candle at both ends
- News binging
- Disconnection from community/meaningful relationships

Lifestyle Stressors

- Burning a candle at both ends
- Bluelight screen exposure (long times on screens)
- Social Media comparison/endless scrolling
- Trying to be all things to all people/people pleasing
- FOMO (lack of downtime for yourself)
- Less than 7 hours of sleep most nights
- Overtraining
- Imbalanced exercise (i.e. doing HIIT/cardio all the time without mixing it up)
- Not talking about your stress (bottling it up)
- Not doing things you love
- Exposure to chemicals in beauty, cleaning and hygiene products
- Plastic tupperware/container use
- Lack of outdoor/nature and fresh air
- Lack of play and fun
- Endlessly Google searching answers to your health questions
- NSAID use (headaches, etc.)
- Birthcontrol and long term medication use
- Disconnection from community/meaningful relationships

Food Stressors

- Frequent coffee/caffeine consumption
- Artificial sweeteners (most commercial stevia included)
- Eating packaged, refined or processed foods
- Low water intake (less than half your bodyweight in ounces)
- Tap water (not filtered)
- Frequent eating out (more than preparing/handling your food)

- High focus on calories, diet plans and food rules
- Lack of Vitamin P (pleasure in foods)
- Low carb intake and/or Low fat intake
- Lack of quality protein (amino acids for your brain)
- Dairy (conventional) consumption
- Grains and "gluten free" processed products (with gluten-cross contaminants)
- Binging/Purging and erratic eating habits
- NOT listening to your gut

Sleep is an often overlooked, but highly valuable "hack" to add to your tool belt for combatting digestive issues. In fact, sleep is part of your digestive process—crucial for elimination and the "full processing" of foods.

Since your body runs off of circadian rhythms (your natural clock), sleeping an adequate amount helps counter stress that otherwise disturbs your digestive process.

In addition, according to ancient and traditional Chinese medicine, the organs in your body are said to run off of a meridian clock—the times of day when particular organs are in "go mode."

Interestingly, your small intestine—the organ where the majority of digestion occurs (6-8 hours per meal)—is most "fired up" in the midday (between 1 and 3 pm) and consequently, this is why many cultures originally began eating a larger mid-day meal as their nourishment.

As for your other organs, your stomach is most "alive" between the hours of 7 am and 9 am, directly following the large intestine hour (5 am to 7 am) and your liver (1 am to 3 am), when your body is eliminating toxins and finishing up your digestion from the previous day during your sleep. (This totally makes sense since you typically "do the doo" when you wake up and then your body is more ready for breakfast and a new day of digesting ahead!).

Generally, an individual with a healthier bowel system will find they poop first thing in the morning shortly after waking (without needing coffee, experiencing diarrhea /loose stools or a difficult time passing stools).

Although your meridian clock may not be 100 percent precise (i.e. a hard start at 5 am and hard stop at 7 am for the large intestine), they *do* reflect that the energy of each organ meridian is strongest for 2 hours in specific cycles, completing a 24-hour cycle every day and each meridian comes into its highest action at a particular time of day.

If or when you fail to get enough sleep, your digestive organs are ultimately unable to be at their fullest potential. In addition, if or when you stay up super late or wake up super early (even if you get "enough" sleep), you throw off your digestive organs' rhythmic dance (particularly for the liver and large intestine—the two organs most responsible for finishing off the elimination process), and set yourself up for bloating, lack of appetite or morning heartburn and nausea as well.

Similar to how your own fitness performance, brain function or energy levels suffer when you don't get "enough" sleep, the *same* thing happens for your digestive system.

So how much sleep do you need?
Generally, most research studies show that between 7 to 9 hours (Hirshkowitz et al, 2015) is the just-right Goldilocks' amount for adequate restoration.

Unfortunately, more than one-third of all Americans get less than 6 hours of sleep, and this amount is associated with the same mental function as an individual who is **legally intoxicated** (Williamson & Feyer, 2000).

Even if you do get *enough* sleep, 50 to 70 million Americans don't have good quality sleep and have some level of sleep difficulty, blood sugar imbalance or chronic disease associated with lack of sleep (CDC, 2017). In other words, the time spent with your head on your pillow does not equivocate to "quality sleep." This may be due to insufficient melatonin levels (the natural body chemical that helps your body sleep) or disrupted circadian rhythms from stress and irregular cortisol levels (stress hormones).

Sleep Better

It's easy to say "get more sleep," but how do you get more quality sleep? Here are 10 essentials for proper and improved sleep hygiene:

1. **Avoid Caffeine (especially later).** Caffeine is a natural stimulant and stressor. If you must drink coffee, keep it to one quality cup in the morning. Cap it after to prevent the disruption of your circadian rhythms and sleep-wake cycles later.

2. **Candle Down.** Turn down the lights at least 1-2 hours before bed to cue up melatonin levels (your sleep-inducing chemicals) and detox from artificial blue light which tells your body to "wake up." In addition, eliminate electronic use during this time, or at the very least, switch electronics to "night mode" along with blue-blocking glasses.

3. **Think Happy Thoughts.** Prepare the body for sweet dreams at night along with your candle-down routine

by: a.) Listening to soothing, relaxing and pleasant sounds or music prior to bed; b.) Spritz your body or lather on some good smelling essential oils (like peppermint and lavender); c.) Reading a leisure book; d.) Think happy thoughts before bed. Instead of worrying about your bank account or some work to-do that won't be resolved tonight, choose to fix your eyes on something you're grateful for or something positive and happy (who knows, maybe a trip to the beach is in your dream future?).

4. **Remove Electronics from Close Proximity of your Bed.** The same thing for electronics goes for the bedroom: Phones, iPads, computers and TV'S all produce light which is a distraction, and also produce electromagnetic frequencies which could interfere with sleep.

5. **Black Out.** Just like blue light is not conducive to winding down at night, any hint of light while we actually sleep is not good, either—light seeping in through the windows from the street lights, your phone or alarm clock. Why? The same as blue light, light in general at night throws our circadian rhythms off (way off). Darken your room at night—completely. Consider blackout curtains if light (even street light) peeps in through your windows, remove red lights from alarm clocks and bright lights from your phone by covering them with a towel.

6. **Comfort is Key.** If you're not comfy, how do you think you're going to sleep? Make sure you have enough room to stretch out, move around and it's the right firmness/softness for you.

7. **Warm Up.** A warm bath or hot shower helps relax your body and muscles before bed.

8. **Then Cool Down.** The body goes to work while you slumber—sleep is when recovery, repair and restoration processes happen (meaning your metabolism fires up!). Knowing this, your body temp naturally rises at night, making a cool home and sleep environment crucial to quality sleep. In addition, a cooler environment induces a drop in your own core temperature, triggering your body's "let's hit the sack" (and sleep through the night) button. The ideal temp? Somewhere around 60-68 degrees—dependent on the individual.

9. **Quiet it Down.** A snoring spouse, the sound of your next door neighbors in their apartment, or background TV noise all disrupt your most optimal sleep. Plug in some ear plugs or download a white-noise app if anything to distill the varying distracting sounds of life happening around you.

10. **Rise with the Sun.** Back in the day, the sun was the natural alarm clock for most folks. Since we no longer sleep outside under the stars (and thanks to Edison and the lightbulb), lights often go on before the sun does. Aim to stick as close to your body's natural circadian rhythms by "rising with the sun." You have to check out this "Natural Sun" Phillips Wake-Up Light Alarm—programmed to mimic the sun rising in your room (no matter what time you need to get up). I can't imagine going back to a regular buzzing alarm clock and feeling like a firefighter going to fight a fire in the middle of the night with my old alarm clock. In addition, check out an app like Sleep Cycle, which analyzes your sleep throughout the night—no matter what time you go to bed—and when it's time to wake up, the app wakes you up in your LIGHTEST sleep phase.

Stress Less Tip: Move It (Just Right)

We all know that exercise is good for us.

Regular exercise has been found to help prevent many chronic diseases and health concerns, from obesity to heart disease, diabetes, metabolic syndrome, cancer, osteoporosis, anxiety, depression, insomnia, dementia, Alzheimer's, and early death.

But did you know, it is also good for digestion?

When we lead sedentary lifestyles or sit for the majority of the day, we *prevent* our digestion and bowels from moving and grooving along, as well as promote more **inflammation in our body** (fun fact: increased sitting has been shown to impair metabolic function and decrease the activity of an enzyme called lipoprotein lipase, or LPL, which is associated with higher triglycerides, lower levels of HDL, and an increased risk of heart disease). Since sitting keeps things super still, if we sit still for too long, the digestive process (and our metabolic function in general) moves slower.

However, keep in mind, the same thing can be said if we move too much.

If we over-train and under-recover, we equally keep our digestion and bowels from moving along. Since exercise is a natural stressor which increases cortisol, when we're exercising, the *last* thing our body wants to do is digest. Couple this with overtraining, and it's as if the body barely gets a break! In fact, a key indicator that you may be overtraining is digestive distress. If you've aligned all the other cards—you're eating well, you're sleeping, drinking clean water and breathing, check in with your movement and training.

The "Goldilocks" approach for exercise is technically recommended at 150 minutes of moderate intensity each week (at least 30 minutes per day 5 days per week).

However, your **Gut Kickstart** protocol is not as black and white, and encourages more than anything *integrating movement into your daily life.*

Gut Kickstart Philosophy: *Move most days of the week with the majority of that being lifestyle movement (mindfully incorporating walking, daily activities and desk breaks).*

If you work a sedentary job, consider "lifestyle movement" as taking stand-breaks every 30-45 minutes to stretch, do 10 pushups, get water, go to the bathroom, or step outside for some fresh air.

As for formal exercise, aim for approximately 3 to 5 days of "formal exercise" of varying intensities and movement (a blend of strength, conditioning and power work), *along* with 2 to 3 days of active rest and movement factored in (i.e. volleyball in the park, a recovery day in the gym, a yoga or dance class, flexibility and mobility training, swimming, playing with your kids in the front yard, doing house and yard work, or simply "chilling out).

Throughout your **Gut Kickstart,** as you become more intuitive with food, you'll also be encouraged to become more intuitive with movement.

Your body was meant to move—not exercise—and it does not know the difference between running on a treadmill or running in a game of tag on the playground. It doesn't know the difference in moving a heavy load of boxes or lifting a barbell over your head 10 times.

According to your innate wiring and physical makeup as well, your body thrives on a balance of all modes of fitness.

Just like it needs water, carbs, fats and proteins, it needs:

- Strength
- Aerobic/Endurance
- Power Bursts
- Flexibility/Rest

Here's a sample "workout" schedule which reflects a balance of movements throughout the week as far as formal exercise goes:

- **Day 1**: Strength Training + Energizer (short conditioning or HIIT)
- **Day 2:** Aerobic Activity or Mobility (does not have to be intense: spinning, running, jogging, walking, hiking, swimming, fitness class, bodyweight movements) or Yoga, Stretching, Pilates
- **Day 3:** Strength Training + Energizer
- **Day 4:** Aerobic Activity or Mobility
- Day 5: Strength Training + Energizer
- **Day 6:** Something Fun, Different, New or Lifestyle Movement (not your usual formal routine in gym, get outside, try a group class, challenge yourself in a new way or go on an adventure)
- **Day 7**: Rest/Active Rest Day

What role does movement play in your life? Do some digging about what activities you currently enjoy, what activities you may be forcing yourself to do (but don't enjoy), and which ones you'd like to do….

Reflection:

1. Your Passions: What "moves" you? What gets you excited or fired up to move?

2. The Good Ol' Days: As a kid, what did you love to do to move your body? Sports? Recess games? Cartwheels?

3. Should Monsters: Do you have any "should" monsters in your life when it comes to exercise or fitness? What are the fitness activities you tell yourself you "should" do? Where did this stem from and is it true?

4. Get Outside the Box: Need some inspiration for getting outside your box? Consider the following activities—circle the ones you'd like to try and put a star by the ones you currently do. Then, by the starred ones, list out at least 2-3 things you like about those activities:

Adventure Racing (Spartan, Warrior Dash, Mud Runs, etc.)
Barre
Baseball
Basketball
Biking (mountain, leisure)
Bodybuilding
Bootcamp
Boxing/Kickboxing
Circuits
Cleaning, Yard Work or other Daily Activities
Cross Country
CrossFit
Dance
Gardening
Golfing
Hiking
Hockey

Jogging
Jump Rope
Kettlebells
Martial Arts
Paddleboarding
Parkour
Pilates
Racquetball
Rollerblading
Rock Climbing/Bouldering
Rowing
Rugby
Running
Sailing Spin/Cycling (indoor)
Skiing
Snorkeling
Spin (outdoors)
Soccer
Surfing
Swimming
Tennis
Track & Field
Trail Running
Triathlons
Volleyball
Wakeboarding
Walking
Water Skiing
Weights/Strength Training
Yoga
Zumba

Bonus: Breathe (Well).
One more essential to add to sleep and movement: Oxygen.

Oxygen is the most vital nutrient you can consume—necessary fuel for all of life, and a vital component of your Gut Kickstart Program. Breathing is a skill that is easily forgotten or misunderstood. Breath is not only important for fueling your daily life, but it is also vital for stressing less and healing your gut. Think about it. When we're stressed, anxious, worried or obsessed with anything (including our own healing), we create tension: Headaches. Furrowed eyebrows. Clenched fists. Pent-up energy.

And where is that tension rooted?

In our gut!

Hello constipation, bloating, indigestion and an irritated gut lining.

What to do about it?

Learn how to breathe and do it often. Incorporating deep breaths into our daily routine—including the morning time, evening wind-down time, and *before meals* is a vital component to your Gut Kickstart.

Here are three steps for **Gut Kickstart Breathing:**

1. **Perfect Your Posture.** Head and chest up. Shoulders back. Poor posture is associated with a "stress response" because if we are sunken inward and we are slumping, we can't get that good abdominal breath.

2. **In Through Your Nose.** Breathe in through your nose and out through your mouth. Inhale for a 5-10 second count, and then release for approximately the same length of time. And make it legit seconds: Count one, 1,000, two, 1,000, three, 1,000, four, 1,000, five, 1,000... Concentrated slow breathing naturally slows down the

body's stress response and signals a "parasympathetic" process (rest).

3. **Belly Breathe**. To ensure you're breathing from your gut—your core—place your hand on your belly and recruit your breaths from your internal fire. Diaphragmatic or "belly" breathing recruits the proper muscles for sustained deep, relaxed breaths for the long haul.

Focus 3: Add in your 5 Daily Gut Love Habits

Now for the real fun: Healing—not just *managing*—your gut health.

There is a difference.

Many times, people go on a "clean diet" thinking it's the cure to all their health woes, including weight loss, bloating, constipation, metabolism and hormone imbalances, autoimmune conditions, anxiety, acne and more.

True, what you eat matters.

However, you and your health are not just what you eat, but also what you actually digest. If your gut suffers from things like bacterial overgrowth, intestinal permeability (leaky gut), dysbiosis (imbalanced bacteria), fungal infection, low stomach acid or food intolerances, then no matter how healthy you eat, you still may not digest (well).

Enter: Your 5 Daily Gut Love Habits.

Five essential daily (game-changing) action steps you can easily incorporate into your everyday busy life.

The best part? Unlike many health habits which take time and repetition before you experience the effects (like building strength or toning in the gym), the positive side effects of these five daily habits are fairly instantaneous. And unlike complicated gut healing protocols or expensive supplements, these 5 Daily Gut Love Habits are all about *minimalism—aiming to do more (gut healing) with less complicated protocols.*

Your 5 Daily Gut Love Habits include:
1. **Hydrate**: Drink half your bodyweight in ounces of water each day (Starting with Warm Lemon Water first thing in the morning)
2. **Boost Stomach Acid**: Consume 1 tbsp. Apple Cider Vinegar in water 1-3 times per day
3. **Gut Kickstart Bugs:** Take a Soil-Based Probiotic + Prebiotic
4. **Taste the Rainbow**: Eat 2-3 Colors with Meals & 2 Servings of Greens Daily
5. **Soothe**: Sip Herbal Tea

By the end of your 28-Day Gut Kickstart, you will incorporate all 5 of these into your daily life. However, if you feel overwhelmed to start, simply begin with **ONE** habit each week through the Reintroduction Phase. Before you know it, they will become second nature.

Here's how they work and a bonus to take them up a notch if you ALREADY do them…

Habit 1: Drink Warm Lemon Water

Consume half your bodyweight in ounces of water each day, beginning with 12-16 ounces of warm water with a spritz of lemon or lemon juice and pinch of sea salt before drinking or eating anything else.

Lemon water is naturally hydrating and alkalizing to the body—helping maintain balance. Drinking water, especially warm water, first thing in the morning can help flush the digestive system and rehydrate the body. After a night spent slumbering and detoxifying, lemon water gives your body an extra boost to flush toxins out the door. Lemon water also naturally boosts stomach acid, setting the stage for a day ahead of healthy digestion.

1. **Bonus 1:** Drink your water in a stainless steel water bottle and opt for clean filtered water.
2. **Bonus 2**: Limit coffee to one 8-ounce cup per day

Coffee 101

Q. Why cut out coffee?! Can I not have it!?
A. Yes and no. Coffee is not innately a bad thing.
Get the facts…

Coffee is Not Hydrating
Many people choose to start their day off with a cup of coffee as their drink of choice, but unfortunately, coffee has the reverse effect on energy and hydration in the long term—naturally dehydrating you. For every 8 ounce cup of coffee you consume, your body needs 12 ounces of water to replenish.

Coffee Depletes Energy
Not only does coffee have a "drying" or dehydrating effect on your body's hydration status, but caffeine, when consumed in excess (i.e. more than one cup/day), can also train your body's cortisol and blood sugar levels to depend on it to function. Since cortisol and blood sugar "thrive" upon stimulants like caffeine and sugar, regular consumption becomes a "crutch" for these two mechanisms. The result? Depleted natural energy *unless* you get your coffee fix.

Coffee is Like Gluten
Coffee (instant coffee in particular) is the most cross-contaminating food with gluten, containing proteins which react with gliadin—the same proteins in gluten-containing foods.

Coffee Feeds Your Gut Bugs
The majority of coffee sold in grocery stores or Starbucks is also cited as one of the moldiest foods we can consume. Coffee beans contain mycotoxins, which can cause poisoning when we ingest too much of them, as well as chronic health conditions. Although mycotoxins are also found in all sorts of other foods, when we drink coffee, we may over-consume these molds to our detriment. Not to mention, your gut bugs LOVE moldy foods. As we continue to feed our gut bugs, we may experience symptoms like constipation, bloating, skin breakouts, seasonal allergies and anxiety.

Pooping After Coffee is Not Natural
Have you ever wondered why you have to go after you drink it OR why you CAN'T go UNLESS you have your coffee?

It's tempting to attribute the effect to caffeine, since that's the ingredient you're going after when you down a cup of coffee. But think about it: Soda doesn't have the same effect. <u>And studies have found that *decaf* coffee</u> (Brown et al, 1990) can have a laxative effect, too.

So why do you have to poop? While some scientists hypothesize that the acidity of coffee may be the reason why at least 30% of all coffee drinkers have to do the "doo" after they eat, think again. The cross-contamination of coffee with gluten, coupled with the stimulating cortisol-inducing effects of caffeine may be more like it. In other words: Pooping after coffee (or ONLY being able to go if you drink coffee) is not natural.

Have Your Cake & Eat it Too

During your 28-Day Reset, you're encouraged to see what your body is capable of without dependence on coffee and caffeine. If you must, take a "balanced" approach to coffee and be a coffee SNOB. Stick to one cup of quality (preferably organic) coffee roast per day with no added sugar. Add a splash of coconut milk, goat's milk kefir, grass-fed ghee or butter or MCT oil for a "creamier" coffee.

As for busting "coffee dependence" headaches? Drink PLENTY of water throughout the day, ensure you're eating proteins and healthy fats with meals and snacks, and consider boosting your body (and brain) with amino acids to help you get "over the hump." Amino acids help balance brain chemicals associated with "caffeine withdrawal" headaches. The most often recommended amino acids to take for caffeine addiction are Tyrosine or DLPA (Phenylalanine). Some do better with one, others do better with the other. Try taking 1,000 mg with breakfast and another 1,000 mg at lunch as you cut out the coffee. Lastly, replace your multiple cups of joe with dandelion tea or Teeccino (herbal tea that tastes like coffee).

Habit 2: Boost Stomach Acid: Consume 1 Tbsp. Apple Cider Vinegar in water

In addition to your morning lemon water, **add 1 tbsp. of Apple cider vinegar to a small glass of 2-4 ounces of water for an extra (healthy) punch of stomach acid to start the day.**

Bonus: Consume with other meals (1-3 times per day).

Can't stomach the taste? Add a drop of pure maple syrup or opt for HCL tablets/capsules (250-700 mg) with Pepsin instead.

Q. What Dose of HCL Should I Take?

A. If you opt for HCL tablets over apple cider vinegar, everyone has a unique dose. To find your custom dose, you can try the "HCL Test." Essentially this involves taking one capsule at a time in one setting until you sense a warmness in your stomach. Warmness means you're taking enough. When you reach that, back your dose down one and you've found your match. Some people need one capsule, others may need to take up to nine capsules of HCL with pepsin. (Note: If you are currently on a PPI drug or pregnant, HCL capsule supplementation is not advised. Opt for apple cider vinegar instead).

The Lowdown on ACV
Apple cider vinegar (ACV) is often referred to as the "magic elixir" of health—cited to help boost metabolism, inhibit allergies and boost immunity! Here are some reasons why.

ACV Boosts Stomach Acid
Hydrochloric Acid. ACV's "superpowers" really all boil down to the gut-healing and enhancing benefits it brings to your digestion through hydrochloric acid.

Hydrochloric acid is the same as found in your stomach acid. Your stomach is the most acidic organ and environment in your body (or at least it should be). Hypochlorhydria or low stomach acid, is a commonly overlooked problem that manifests in signs and symptoms like acid reflux, heartburn, burping, gas, bloating, chronic constipation, IBS, brittle nails and hair, nutrient deficiencies, nausea after eating, AND other health related conditions (like a slow metabolism, allergies and illness). Hydrochloric acid is necessary for proper digestion to occur.

ACV Kills Bad Bacteria
One of the chief roles of stomach acid is to inhibit bacterial overgrowth. It's powerful acidic forces help keep your stomach sterile

and break down food from larger particles into nutrients which can begin their journey down your small intestine and large intestine. At a pH of three or less, which is the normal pH of the stomach, most bacteria can't survive for more than 15 minutes, but when stomach acid is low and the pH of your stomach rises above five, bacteria begin to thrive.

ACV Helps Digest Protein & Prevent Abdominal Pain
ACV to the rescue! ACV is particularly helpful for breaking down proteins—one of the most complex nutrients to digest. In fact, many individuals who follow a vegetarian and vegan diet, as well as pregnant women, complain that protein hurts their stomach. Low stomach acid is more than likely at the real reason why.

Habit 3: Take a Soil Based Probiotic & Prebiotic

Take a soil-based probiotic every morning and evening, and one prebiotic serving once per day.

Bonus:

Eat 1-2 Servings of probiotic & prebiotic-rich foods each day.
Add 1-2 Digestive enzymes with meals to assist in complete digestion.

Probiotic & Prebiotic 101

All long-term gut healing protocols should include both probiotics and prebiotics for *optimal* results—two natural substances you can find in supplements and foods.

The Lowdown on Probiotics
We often hear probiotics are "good for our gut," but no one ever really tells us why beyond saying they are "good gut bacteria." True, probiotics do help boost gut bacteria, but they also:

- Protect your gut lining
- Influence the amount of antioxidants in your body
- Impact your brain health (balance your mood, improve concentration and function)
- Guard against stress in your gut (from bad foods to low stomach acid)
- Fight inflammation
- Fight off SIBO
- Limit carbohydrate malabsorption (aid in FODMAP intolerance)
- Aid in nutrient absorption
- Reduce histamines (allergies)
- Guard against limit gastric or intestinal pathogens (parasites, fungi and viruses)

Way more than just giving you "good gut bacteria!"

The Low Down on Prebiotics
While probiotics DO get a lot of hype in the media, prebiotics are actually arguably MORE important and necessary. In fact, taking probiotics ALONE does NOT "boost your gut bacteria" or make more in your gut. **Prebiotics are fiber-based foods and supplements which *feed* probiotics in the first place.**

Probiotics need prebiotics in order to "stick" in your gut and research has shown that higher intakes of prebiotic foods can increase numerous probiotic microorganisms. In addition, prebiotics help increase stool regularity, improve your brain-gut (mood) connection and lower inflammation.

Probiotics & Prebiotics: How They Work Together
For a long time, we've thought that taking probiotics is like putting gas into your car tank—you fill it up and there's more gas.

But it doesn't work that way. Instead, probiotics only serve as "maintainers" or regulators of the "good" gut bacteria you ALREADY have in your body—but they don't necessarily produce more. Sure, your body certainly welcomes probiotics, and probiotics do help keep your current healthy bacteria operating at their peak, but you don't get MORE or increase the numbers of "good gut bacteria" in your gut. Moreover, if you STOP taking your probiotics, your "healthy gut" bacteria no longer has something else helping it out to stay "healthy" *unless* you take and eat a prebiotic.

Prebiotics **DO** increase the beneficial bacteria because they provide food for those beneficial species in the first place. When you consume prebiotics, you help multiply your probiotics so you can increase beneficial bacteria over time.

The Bonus? Even if you stop taking your prebiotic, those probiotic numbers would stay increased (provided you eat enough prebiotic fiber to feed those bacteria in your daily diet).

CHOOSE THE RIGHT PROBIOTIC & PREBIOTIC FOR YOU)

So how do you choose the "right" probiotic and prebiotic for you? Not all probiotics and prebiotics are created equal. Generally, you get what you pay for, but there is more to it than that.

For instance, for a probiotic to perform its necessary function, it must naturally survive the stomach's harsh environment and arrive at the intestines alive. A true probiotic is designed by nature and is a species found in our environment, as well as in our digestive system. Approximately 90-95 percent of probiotic products on shelves today do NOT meet these criteria, based on studies.

Probiotics 101

When choosing your probiotic and prebiotic supplements, here's what you need to know:

There are 4 main types of probiotics:

- **Lactobacillus Strains** (including Lactobacillus acidophilus, Lactobacillus plantarum, Lactobacillus reuteri, Lactobacillus rhamnosus, and Lactobacillus salivarius)
  - ▷ Most common type of bacteria found in your gut already
  - ▷ Most common type found in supplements on shelves, however also most commonly falsely advertised supplements s as well
  - ▷ Best sources: Fermented foods (veggies, dairy and meats)
  - ▷ Can cause symptoms of bloating, nausea, loose stools and/or constipation in individuals with underlying GI dysfunction (SIBO, parasites, anti-fungal, etc.)
- **Bifidobacteria species**
  - ▷ Best sources: Fermented veggies, dairy and meats
  - ▷ Can help prevent and treat GI disorders and diseases (colon cancer, GI infections, diarrhea, etc.)
- **Saccharomyces boulardii**
  - ▷ Found in kefir, kombucha, fermented veggies, fermented dairy and fermented soy (natto, tofu)
  - ▷ Great for IBS and diarrhea/loose stools
  - ▷ Reduces *difficile* infection
- **Soil-based organisms (SBOs)**
  - ▷ Normal "residents" of a healthy gut

- ▷ Best tolerated supplements amongst the majority of people
- ▷ Found in dirt from healthy soil on organic produce and in supplements
- ▷ Beneficial for chronic diarrhea, iBS, chronic fatigue syndrome, diabetes
- ▷ Avoid Bacillus Anthracis, Bacillus cereus, Bacillus licheniformis
- ▷ Bacillus clausii and Bacillus subtilis are the most widely studied and effective strains to date

Q. Which one do I choose?!
A. As a baseline supplement, opt for a **broad-spectrum soil-based or spore-based probiotic** (i.e. containing more than one strain of bacteria). Note: Make sure your probiotics list the strains. If they don't, you already know it's no good.

Soil-based organisms resemble the healthy bacteria in the gut most similar to the bacteria humans had in their guts thousands of years ago—when they lived off the food from the land. Food which was nutrient-dense and diverse. Also, soil-based organisms tend to be well-tolerated by most people.

Probiotic Brand Supplement Suggestions:

- Primal Probiotics
- Seed Daily Probiotic
- MegaSpore Biotic
- Garden of Life Primal Defense Ultra (contains some some soil-based strains, but also lactic acid bacteria strains; avoid if you have SIBO or elevated D-Lactate)
- AOR3
- FloraMyces

Best Probiotic Foods:
Sauerkraut
Fermented Veggies (carrots, beets, cucumber relish, dill pickles, etc.)
Pickled Veggies (no added sugar or additives)
Fermented Salsa
Fermented Horseradish
Goat's Milk Yogurt & Kefir
Coconut Kefir
Water Kefir
Coconut Yogurt (no additives)
Low-Sugar Kombucha (2-3 grams per serving)
Beet Kvass
Kimchi
Fermented Tofu, Miso & Natto (not processed)

Ways to Eat Probiotic Foods:
- Eat 2-3 forkfuls of sauerkraut or fermented veggies straight from the jar
- Use kefir (goats milk, coconut, water) as the base of a smoothie
- Add blueberries to kefir or full-fat yogurt (goat's milk, coconut) and eat as a dessert
- Sip 2-4 oz. of a low-sugar Kombucha (max 2-3 grams per serving)
- Drink beet kvass

Q. Why not lactic acid bacteria probiotic supplements?
A. Unfortunately, the MAJORITY of probiotics sold in stores contain lactic acid bacteria. However, you're more than likely wasting your money on most of these since (a.) they often don't contain the strains of bacteria they claim, as they are easily processed, heated or destroyed in production, and (b.) your body often already has enough of many of these lactic acid strains—similar to many of the bacteria which end up in your poop.

The Exception:
If you can't tolerate fermented foods, there are a select amount of quality lactic acid bacteria and Bifidobacteria probiotics out there. Look for supplements from a quality manufacturer that require refrigeration and contain a variety of strains…. Some recommendations include: Therabiotic Complete (Klaire Labs), VSL#3.

Prebiotics 101

Like probiotics, the world of prebiotics can be overwhelming.

Prebiotics come in both supplement and starch form, and there are three main types of prebiotics:

- **Soluble Fiber**
    - ▷ Best sources: Partially hydrolyzed guar gum powder, glucomannan powder, acacia fiber powder, citrus pectin, cooked vegetables (carrots, butternut squash, squashes)
    - ▷ Best tolerated by patients with gut issues in general because they're not FODMAPs and they tend to have a soothing effect on the digestive tract

- **Non-starch polysaccharides**
  - ▷ Best whole-food sources: Mushrooms (reishi, shiitake, maitake) seaweed, algae, onion, garlic, asparagus)
  - ▷ Least well-tolerated by those with IBS and SIBO, because the majority of these are FODMAP foods (including inulin and FOS (fructooligosaccharides), larch arabinogalactan, galactooligosaccharides, and beta-glucan; common gut-irritating and FODMAP foods including wheat, beans, peas, chickpeas, grains, raw apples/pears, onions, broccoli, commercial yogurts, dairy)
- **Resistant Starch**
  - ▷ Best sources: Cooked and cooled sweet potatoes/potatoes, green-tipped bananas/plantains, parboiled white rice (cooked and cooled), legumes
  - ▷ Increases the concentration of short-chain fatty acids like butyrate and propionate (which aid in digestion)
  - ▷ Shown to protect against colon cancer, improve metabolic health, reduce fasting blood sugar and body weight, and improve insulin sensitivity
  - ▷ Help with sleep and mood (insomnia, depression, anxiety)
  - ▷ Can limit SIBO and bacterial overgrowth
  - ▷ Aid in mineral and nutrient absorption

Q. Which prebiotic do I choose?!

As far as supplements go, in clinical practice, partially hydrolyzed guar gum and glucomannan powder tend to be the best tolerated amongst most people, and for real-food sources, resistant starches like cooked and cooled sweet potatoes/ potatoes, green-tipped bananas and plantains, as well as soluble fibers (cooked carrots, cooked squashes) Choose one prebiotic supplement to take with your probiotics away from food, and incorporate colorful prebiotic foods into your diet (i.e. starchy tubers, veggies and fruits).

Prebiotic Supplements:
Partially Hydrolyzed Guar Gum* (preferred choice)
Acacia Fiber
Unmodified potato starch
Glucomannan powder
Psyllium husk powder
Modified Citrus Pectin
Food sources: Eat throughout your week

Prebiotic Foods*:
Asparagus (al dente)
Banana (green-tipped)
Cooked & Cooled Sweet Potatoes/Potatoes
Cooked & Cooled Parsnips, Winter Squash, Carrots, Squashes
Dandelion greens
Eggplant
Endive
Garlic
Raw Honey
Jerusalem artichokes
Jicama
Kefir
Leeks

Legumes
Onions
Peas
Plantains (green-tipped)
Radicchio
Mushrooms (reishi, shiitake and maitake)
Nutritional Yeast
Potato Starch or Plantain Starch
Seaweed/Algae (Beta-glucan, or β-glucan—a soluble fiber)

*Not all fibers in foods have prebiotics (grain fibers in particular are indigestible, making the fiber in them negative).

Ways to Eat Prebiotic Foods:
- Mix psyllium husk powder with unmodified potato starch in water, unsweetened almond milk, or add to a smoothie
- Add glucomannan powder to water, almond milk, or a smoothie
- Make plantain "pancakes" with green-tipped plantains, plantain flour, or potato starch
- Eat half of a green-tipped banana dipped in coconut butter or raw nut butter as a snack
- Add a cooked and cooled sweet potato or regular potato to your dinner
- Add artichoke hearts to your salad
- Cook with fresh onions

How to Take Them:
In general, probiotics are best taken with your prebiotics on an otherwise empty stomach.

For maximum absorption, aim to take a probiotic supplement once in the morning and once at night, *along* with your prebiotic once per day—preferably away from meals (at least 15-30 minutes before or after).

Integrate Slowly

As "healing" or die-off reactions happen, some people may experience GI upset, increased gas and/or bloating as they incorporate these new supplements (generally, this improves in a few days). Start slowly with the amount of both probiotics and prebiotics you take, and gradually increase the dose of both as tolerated, based on symptoms of gut distress. For instance,

- Probiotics: Take one capsule daily for seven days, then increase to one capsule twice daily.
- Prebiotic powders: Start with ½ tsp-1 tsp per day, or every other day, and increase in ½ tsp amounts every 3-4 days untils one full serving is achieved
- Take away from food, between meals (at least 15-30 minutes before or after).

Q. Can't I just get all my probiotics and prebiotics from foods and supplements?

A. It's true, fermented foods and real-food fibers have many advantages over commercial probiotic products. For instance, the concentration of probiotic organisms is significantly higher in some fermented foods. However, for your Gut Kickstart, BOTH food and supplements are important and useful in a treatment plan.

While fermented foods provide huge amounts of lactic acid bacteria, probiotic supplements include other varieties of bacteria, too, which may not be found in all fermented foods you eat. Probiotic supplements can be used to achieve more specific gut-healing goals—such treating constipation or diarrhea. In addition, some people simply don't tolerate fermented foods well, especially if they are amine intolerant or histamine or tyramine intolerant.

Habit 4: Eat 2-3 Colors with Meals + 2 Servings of Greens Daily

Aim to include 2-3 different colors at **each meal,** including 2 servings of green veggies SOMEWHERE in your day.

As you build your meals upon proteins, fats and carbs—particularly color rich veggies or "phytonutrients" (the colorful components of plants that are powerful defenders of health)—your gut will become Popeye strong.

Although some foods may still not sit well with you (such as cruciferous vegetables or FODMAP fruits), aim to eat in abundance as many **colorful** foods as possible. Colorful foods are where all your fibers, vitamins and minerals are—particularly prebiotic fibers, found in many starchy tubers and root veggies.

For instance, deep blue or purplish blueberries contain Quercetin and anthocyanin-nutrients that boost brain health. Bright orange beta-carotene in sweet potatoes and carrots is connected to ovulation and healthy hormones. Lutein, a yellow-like compound in foods like kale, enhances vision and eye health.

Additionally, phytonutrient (color) rich foods contain more **antioxidants**—compounds that fight off free radicals and toxins (that our leaky gut and liver often have to fight off as well).

These carb-based foods are NOT the enemy.

Carbs—especially plant sources like veggies, starchy veggies and some fruits— help improve digestion through pre-biotics and fiber that help push food through the digestive tract. Pair along with healthy fats and a moderate amount of building-block proteins for max absorption.

How many should you get? Aim for 6-12 servings of plant foods every day.

Note: 9 out of 10 Americans do NOT eat the recommended serving of veggies every day.

One serving equates to one cup of leafy greens or a half cup serving (fist-sized) of other veggies or piece of fruit. (The good news? You can essentially get four to five servings of plant foods just in a lunchtime salad).

Go for the rainbow! Here are some ideas:

Red Foods

- Apples
- Beans (Adzuki, Kidney, Red)
- Beets
- Bell pepper
- Blood oranges
- Cranberries
- Cherries
- Grapefruit (pink)
- Goji berries
- Grapes
- Onions
- Plums
- Pomegranate
- Potatoes
- Radicchio
- Radishes
- Raspberries
- Strawberries
- Sweet red peppers
- Rhubarb
- Rooibos tea
- Tomato
- Watermelon

Blue Foods

- Bell pepper
- Berries (blue, black, boysenberries, huckleberries, marionberries)
- Cabbage
- Carrots
- Cauliflower
- Prunes
- Raisins
- Eggplant
- Figs
- Grapes
- Kale
- Olives
- Plums
- Potatoes
- Rice (black, purple

Yellow Foods

Apple
Asian pears
Banana
Bell peppers
Ginger root
Lemon
Pineapple
Potatoes
Starfruit
Succotash
Summer squash

White/Tan Foods

Apples
Applesauce
Cauliflower
Cocoa
Coconut
Dates
Garlic
Ginger
Jicama
Mushrooms
Nuts (almonds, cashews, pecans, walnuts)
Onions
Pears
Sauerkraut
Seeds (flax, hemp, pumpkin, sesame, sunflower)
Shallots

Green Foods

Apples
Artichoke
Asparagus
Avocado
Bamboo sprouts
Bean sprouts
Bell peppers
Bitter melon
Bok choy
Broccoli
Broccolini
Brussels sprouts
Cabbage
Celery
Cucumbers
Edamame/Soybeans
Green beans
Green peas

Green tea
Greens (arugula, beet, chard, collard, dandelion, kale, lettuce, mustard, spinach, turnip)
Limes
Okra
Olives
Pears
Snow peas
Watercress
Zucchini

Orange Foods

Apricots
Bell pepper
Cantaloupe
Carrots
Mango
Nectarine
Orange
Papaya
Persimmons
Pumpkin
Squash (acorn, buttercup, butternut, winter)
Sweet potato
Tangerines
Turmeric root
Yams

Incorporate variety and experiment with different fibrous foods that may work better with your body. Here are some ways to get more phytonutrients into your daily diet:

- Try one new plant food every week
- Throw some on top of a salad
- Use veggie-based and mushroom-based sauces
- Pre-slice veggies when you get home from the store to make it easy to use them
- Switch from pasta to spaghetti squash or zucchini noodles
- Choose fruit for dessert
- Stock up on some frozen veggies and berries for in-a-pinch moments when yours have gone bad
- Choose veggies and fruits that are dark and rich in color
- Shop in season
- Vary up your starches—butternut, carrots, sweet potatoes, beets, etc.
- Add lemon, grapefruit or mint and cucumber to water

- Make dishes with veggie variety (soups, stir fries, hashes, etc.)
- Use the fruits and vegetables that go bad faster first. Save hardier varieties for later in the week.

Gut Kickstart Tip: Banish Veggie Bloat & Constipation

Veggies are great for you, but sometimes they can also make us feel bloated or constipated—especially if we have underlying bacterial overgrowth or food intolerances. If this is you, consider prepping your veggies in "digestive friendly" ways, including:

- Pan sautéing in healthy fat
- Steaming or roasting with healthy fat
- Chopping
- Pureeing
- Peeling
- Adding greens to casseroles, soups or smoothies
- Experimenting with trying a low-FODMAP approach while you work on healing your gut

Habit 5: Soothe

Sip one cup of herbal tea before bed every night to boost digestion and/or drink 1 cup of bone broth or meat broth daily to soothe your gut lining

Types to try:
Ginger
Peppermint
Fennel
Dandelion

Herbs Do a Body Good

Long before Tums, Ibuprofen, Pepto Bismol or Colace, people used different foods and herbs for to easing digestion and assisting in elimination.

Common foods which are gut loving superstars include:

- Bone Broth
- Sauerkraut & Fermented Veggies
- Grass-fed Yogurt
- Coconut Oil, Ghee & Extra Virgin Olive Oil
- Prebiotic Fibers—like Green-Tipped Bananas, Plantains, Onions, Cooked & Cooled Sweet Potatoes
- Garlic
- Celery
- Cinnamon
- Turmeric
- Herbs—like oregano, dandelion, cilantro, basil, mint and ginger

Herbs are nature's gut healing agents. They help speed digestion up by increasing the digestive secretions in your stomach which help break down food quickly and effectively. Herbs also warm up digestion—helping reduce gas and bloating, stimulating bile flow (waste), and decreasing abdominal pain.

How to consume them? Aside from tea, use fresh herbs in your cooking to season meat and veggies, chew on a piece of raw ginger, throw them into smoothies, or diffuse essential oils in the air (yes, clean air can also help promote healthy digestion).

Summary

We covered a lot of ground. As a refresher, your 5 Daily Gut Love Habits include:

1. **Hydrate**: Drink Warm Lemon Water first thing in the morning
2. **Boost Stomach Acid**: Consume 1 tbsp. Apple Cider Vinegar in water 1-3 times per day
3. **Reset Your Gut Bugs:** Take a Soil-Based Probiotic + Prebiotic
4. **Taste the Rainbow**: Eat 2-3 Colors with Meals & 2 Servings of Greens Daily
5. **Soothe:** Sip herbal tea or 1 cup meat or bone broth daily.

Little things make a big difference, and during your 28-Day Gut Kickstart, we're aiming for healing, not just managing gut health.

Next Level

Want to take your 5 Daily Gut Love Habits to the next level?
See the Resources section for additional Supplemental & Lifestyle Supports, as well as "Cheat Sheet" Gut Healing protocols for every "ailment" under the sun—from gas and bloating, to constipation, SIBO, allergies and everything in between.

Phase 3: Reintroduction & Maintenance

Let the Reintroduction Phase begin!

After 28 days of "resetting" your palate and giving your gut a break to heal, Phase 3 officially starts now: experimenting and reintroducing with any foods you've been wondering how they affect you, AND customizing a way of eating as well as supplements that work for you.

The best part? Plans and diet rules are gone! You are going to practice Intuitive & Mindful Eating Skills to help you figure out what's best for YOUR BODY—instead of me telling you what to do.

What is Intuitive & Mindful Eating?

I'm glad you asked!

Intuitive & Mindful Eating 101

Intuitive & mindful eating is all about listening to your body and trusting your gut.

They are natural human skills you were born knowing how to do.

Intuitively…

You cried when you were hungry. Turned your head away from your mom or your bottle when you were full. You slept when you were tired. Played when you had energy.

And Mindfully…
You were 100% present and connected with how you felt, and mindful to listen to what your body needed

Unfortunately, you grew up and intuitive and mindful eating became extremely hard to practice—especially with protocols, food rules and the "shoulds" and "shouldn'ts" of modern day culture.

BUT imagine…What would it be like to:

- To eat when you're hungry and *know* when you're full?
- To eat a big hearty salad with lots of avocado, fresh herbs, juicy tomatoes and salmon one day, and to eat a grilled cheese and homemade chicken noodle soup the next on a cold day.
- To eat a few bites too many of your mom's homemade spaghetti (because it tastes really good and you enjoy the comfort of a home cooked meal), or to choose a smoothie or broth one evening for dinner instead of a large meal because you ate a later lunch that day?
- To crave chocolate—and allow yourself to eat some chocolate; or to crave a crisp apple, and eat the apple?
- To STOP thinking about your next meal, and to be fully present with your work, your blog, your painting, your to-do list, the book or podcast you're listening to, or anything else at hand?

Oh my, how the tables would turn.

This week and beyond, you're encouraged to begin honing in on your own intuitive eating skills.

Here are 4 ways:

1: Tune it Out
First things first, if you want to truly get back to your natural language of listening to your own body—and less to rules—be pro-active in tuning out the noise and distractions. Your thoughts are not always true. Repeat: Your thoughts are not always true. Use your Reintroduction Phase to experiment with some new foods and let your body determine how you feel more than your brain.

2: Continue to Love Your Gut (Health)
Continue to support your gut with a healthy baseline of probiotics, prebiotics, apple cider vinegar and digestive enzymes as needed. In addition, consider doing any additional testing of your gut, now that you have a "clean slate" to truly assess how you feel.

3: Ask
One simple question to ask yourself (and your gut) when the question of "what to eat" or "what to do to workout" or even how to spend your time: "How do I feel?"

Closing your eyes can often help here, and even placing your hand on your gut. Ask your body (and your head and your heart) what it is you truly want. (And have no judgment). A balanced body is not ALWAYS going to say chocolate…or ALWAYS going to say salads…or ALWAYS going to say coffee…or ALWAYS going to say CrossFit…or ALWAYS going to say "sit on the couch!" A balanced body needs yin and yang. And the more you practice this art…the more trusting you will become.

4: Go With Your Gut Feeling
Often times, you ALREADY know your answer. Or your gut does. Your intuition. Trust it. Challenge yourself—even for one meal, or one day—to simply "listen to your gut."

How do I reintroduce foods?

The key here is: One at a time.

Here's a simple step-by-step guide for incorporating foods back in one-by-one after your 28 Day Reset.

Step 1: One at a Time
Instead of eating several different reintroduction foods in the same setting or day, it's best to gradually reintroduce foods one by one. That way you know how one food affects you, if at all differently, from another.

Step 2: A Little Bit Will Do You
For whichever food you choose incorporate just a little bit at a time. Not a full serving at once. A few bites on day one, followed by a little more on the following days.

Step 3: Give it 3 Days
Eat a little bit of that reintroduction food 3 days in a row to give your body time to readjust to something new and re-acclimate.

Step 4: Evaluate
How do you feel? Any signs or symptoms you notice? (skin breakouts, allergies, upset tummy, etc.). Go with your gut, and move into experimenting with other foods if you like

How do I know if a food doesn't work for my body?

As you begin Experimenting & Reintroducing foods, the topic of Food Intolerances is a given—recognizing foods that don't agree with you. Gut problems often go hand-in-hand with food intolerances—certain foods that trigger an inflammatory response inside your gut.

The tricky thing? You may NOT always FEEL food intolerances in your gut.

In fact, common "signs" of food intolerances include things like skin breakouts, acne, ADD/ADHD, brain fog, headaches, anxiety, joint pain, nutrient deficiencies, hormonal imbalances, and other non-gut-related symptoms.

We can eat foods for years and suffer the "consequences" without ONCE attributing it to the foods we eat.

To make things even more complicated, we OFTEN crave foods we are intolerant to. If you find that you crave certain foods that don't always make you feel the best (i.e. headaches, heart palpitations, bloating, loose stools), but continue to want to eat them anyways, there IS a reason: Hungry bacteria.

Your (bad) gut bugs LOVE feeding off foods that ferment in your gut, and will signal to your body to eat more of them to make them happy.

This is the reason why you may crave that bag of nuts or sugar time and time again—even though you always feel constipated after you eat them, or the reason why you continue to eat sweet potatoes, several times per day, even though bloating happens time and time again.

Your gut bugs like them.

Allergies vs. Intolerances

It's important to understand that intolerance is not the same as allergy. Food allergies are IgE- mediated, whereas intolerances are IgG- or IgA-mediated.

IgE, IgG and IgA refers to different types of immunoglobulins or "antibodies" that are part of our immune system, and are produced in response to things we come in contact with on a daily basis.

Our bodies create antibodies to foreign substances like bacteria and viral cells, but can also respond to foods, dust, dander, and pollen. Antibodies help the body trigger an immune system response to fight against foreign invaders.

However, when we have TOO many antibodies, this can cause either:

1. An immediate allergic reaction (IgE response), such as watery eyes, diarrhea, hives and difficulty breathing; OR
2. A food sensitivity reaction (IgA and IgG response). Food sensitivity reactions are usually more delayed (several hours to days) and encompass a variety of symptoms not always directly connected to gut health, like:
   - Brain fog or Headaches
   - Joint pain
   - Blood sugar imbalances (hypo/hyperglycemia)
   - ADD/ADHD
   - Intestinal discomfort
   - Rashes & skin breakouts

Food allergies are most commonly diagnosed in childhood by an allergist using a skin prick, oral testing, blood test or an oral food challenge.

Food intolerances, on the other hand, are RARELY assessed in conventional medicine practices. Due to their "silent" and less overt symptoms (that look like other diseases and imbalances), food intolerances often go undiagnosed.

So how do you know if you have food intolerances?
Blood testing, hair testing and saliva testing are the current standard methods of testing for food intolerances.

However, it's important to realize: Not all food intolerance tests are created equal….especially testings often sold online or in a nutritionist's office including:

- ALCAT
- MRT
- ELISA

These testing methods are NOT valid because:

1. They have not shown consistent and replicable results from sample to sample;
2. Labs do not always test for foods in the form they are consumed in (i.e. raw vs. cooked). Many labs for test for the raw versions of foods alone (eggs, chicken, broccoli, etc.), without regard that you actually may eat those foods cooked. Cooking changes the proteins in foods, so any "positive" results may not be 100% accurate;

Is there another option other than food intolerance text?
YES!

It's called "experimenting" (exactly what you are doing this week)!

In addition, if you choose to run a food intolerance test, you want a test that tests for both IgG and IgA antibodies, as well as the raw and cooked versions of the foods being tested (instead of raw chicken or potato) and that has been clinically validated. Cyrex Labs is the most respected food intolerance testing lab to date. However, if food intolerance lab testing is not in the cards, consider trying the Coca's Pulse Test you learned about during your Prep Week.

Coca's Pulse Test Refresher

The Coca's Pulse Test is an at-home nutritional therapy evaluation that helps determine any "allergic tension" an individual may have. Here's how to do it.

- Collect any foods you'd like to test for possible food allergies (ex. oatmeal, bread, nuts, cheese, rice, tomato, apples, eggs, etc.).
- Take your resting pulse x 1 minute while seated and relaxed.
- Then place the test food in your mouth.
- Salivate it for 30 seconds.
- Retake your resting pulse x 1 minute while seated and relaxed.

If your pulse changes by six beats or more, it is indicative of "allergic tension." You can perform this for as many suspected foods as you like, and of course, be on the lookout for other markers.

What happens after the Reintroduction?

Maintenance! ("Your Sweet Spot")

By this stage in the game, there's a good chance you've discovered the foods that do (and don't) agree with you and your gut, as well as the lifestyle game changers (like sleep and workout habits) that influence how you feel.

This is where you "do you"--your personal protocol.

You just eat food and live your life, ultimately in ways that make you feel good inside and out.

If it helps, create a "Bill of Rights" or your own list of "rules" to lead and live by--go with your gut.

CHAPTER 8

The Secret Sauce (Gut Love)

You will not fully heal, until you learn to (show gut) love…to yourself.

While you can experiment with how different foods make you feel, run lab tests, pop probiotics and digestive enzymes, and see what coffee enemas do for "cleansing your system," nothing is going to push the needle towards healing all of you like love—authentic self-love.

No, not narcissism, self-obsession or cheesy affirmations,, but genuine compassion, nourishment with real foods, self-care, self-respect and patience with your healing process.

Defining "Gut Love"

What does "gut love" mean to you?

According to Webster's love is…
    (noun) "an intense feeling of deep affection."
    (noun) "a person or thing that one loves."
    (verb) "to feel deeply about someone or something."

Plain and simple, love is a feeling, an act, and a particular affection for something (like yourself, or your own health and self-care) which stems directly from your inner core—your gut feelings.

If you have a difficult time wrapping your head around the concept of "love" and how "gut love" (self-love, love for others, and loving what you do) plays into your overall gut healing process, consider this:

What is the opposite of love?

Hate.

Tension. Stress. Frustration. Annoyance.

When you feel hate, what do you think happens to your body, your heart and your mind?

You get tense. You stress. You furrow your brow, clench your fists and your teeth, clench your stomach. You tighten up and get knots in your stomach. If we do not love, we're left with hate, or at the very least, unrest (stress, tension and turmoil inside and out).

As humans, we are all born with natural instincts for survival. When our survival instincts feel threatened (i.e. stress, hate, disconnection from ourselves), our natural instincts respond accordingly—we fight for survival (often leading to extra mental and physical stress inflicted on our body in response).

Hello gut bugs, constipation, bloating, dysbiosis, ulcers, headaches, bloating, skin flare ups and breakouts!

On the other hand, when we love from the center and core of who we are—and when we love BIG (with an open heart of genuine self-love and self-acceptance), then healing is made even MORE possible.

What will "gut love" look like for you in your own life?

Still stumped?

Well, how do you show love for other people—say a good friend or your significant other?

- You think about them.
- You check in with them.
- You spend time with them.
- You let them know.
- You give them your attention and focus.
- You care for them.
- You pray for them or think good thoughts for them.
- You enjoy them.
- You feel refreshed by them.
- You connect with them.

Ultimately, love makes us care.

And that is what "gut love" is all about—caring for yourself enough to love yourself, even when you don't fully feel at peace or accepting of yourself yet.

Repeat after me:

"This is my body, my health, my life and my heart. I love and accept my body, my health, my life and my heart—just as I am."

When you believe that at your core, gut healing is yours for the taking.

CHAPTER 9

Get Started: Your 28-Day Gut Kickstart

Get it? Got it? Good. Improved gut health is yours for the taking! So what's next? Getting started!

Here's a refresher check-list of each of the 3 Phases of your Gut Kickstart, along with tons of resources in the back of this book.

28-Day Gut Kickstart Works

Your Gut Kickstart is divided into 3 phases:

Phase 1 (Week 1): Prep Week
Phase 2 (Weeks 2-5): 28-Day Reset Phase
Phase 3 (Weeks 6+): Reintroduction & Maintenance Phase (finding your "sweet spot" and living out your new "norm")

Phase 1 (Week 1): Prep Week

Prior to beginning your 28-Day Gut Kickstart, use these seven days to:

Assess

Conduct additional assessments along with your food log, and/or any additional (optional) lab tests:**

Keep a Prep Days Food Log

In addition, during your Prep Week, it's highly recommended you keep a 3-7 day Mindful Food Log. Refer back to Phase 1 for the details of how to keep your Mindful Food Log.

Get Prepped

- Grocery shop for necessary foods
- Wean yourself off of your "old" habits (ie. multiple cups of coffee, eating on the go not sleeping enough, etc.)
- Purchase your supplements (probiotic, prebiotic, digestive enzymes*)

Baseline Supplement Recommendations

- Apple Cider Vinegar or HCL Capsules (600-700 mg HCL/pepsin)
- Herbal Tea of choice
- Soil Based Probiotic
- Prebiotic Fiber
- Digestive Enzymes (Optional)

Bonus: Take it to the Next Level: 24-48 Hour Gut Kickstart Cleanse.

Already been eating an anti-inflammatory AIP, GAPS, SCD or other gut-healing diet? You have the option during the initial 24-48 hours of your kickstart to kick it off with a 24-48 hour Reset Cleanse. This initial protocol is a "reset" for your kickstart in order to help you sift through any foods you may currently be eating daily that still don't agree with you, as well as to encourage variety when you reintroduce other foods during the 28 days. Use a 24-48 hour Gut Kickstart Cleanse with easy-to-digest purees, foods, soups and smoothies to wipe the slate clean.

The 28 Day Gut Kickstart

24-48 Hour Gut Kickstart Cleanse Foods to Eat

Easy to Digest Foods:
- Fermented Foods (1-2 servings; no dairy)
- Bone Broth/Meat Stock & Soups/Stews
- Low-Sugar Vegetable Juices (Beet, Carrot, Green Fresh Juice, no added fruits or sugar)
- Dark Leafy Greens, sauteed in coconut oil or ghee
- Stewed or Cooked Veggies (Low FODMAP, Zucchini, Yellow Squash, Asparagus, Green Beans; no cruciferous)
- Minimal Fruits (Low FODMAP)
- Healthy Fats: Coconut Oil, Coconut Butter, Avocado Oil, Ghee, Coconut Yogurt, Coconut Flakes, Extra Virgin Olive Oil, Olives
- Proteins: Wild Caught Fatty Fish; Stewed Meats/Chicken (Shredded Pastured/Organic Chicken, Grass-fed Roast and Crockpot or Stewed Meats)
- Low Sugar Smoothies (1 fruit only, additive-free proteins or powders)

**Note on Lab Testing:
Lab testing is not required or necessary for your 28-day protocol, but if you want to get to the bottom of your health with more clinical insights, consult with a skilled, knowledgeable healthcare provider to run necessary gut lab work to establish a baseline of where you are starting. (Refer back to Chapter 7A for all lab test recommendations).

Functional Medicine Practitioner Directories

Kresser Institute Practitioners:
https://kresserinstitute.com/directory/

Institute for Functional Medicine:
https://www.ifm.org/find-a-practitioner/

Functional Medicine Coaching Academy
https://www.functionalmedicinecoaching.org

Phase 2 (Weeks 2-5): 28-Day Reset

Now you're ready to dive in! The 2 essentials of your 28-Day Reset are:

1. **Eat Real Food* & Drink Clean Water (See your Resources for your complete food list and meal ideas)**
2. **Add ONE of your 5 Daily Gut Love Habits Each Week**
   - Week 1: Drink half your bodyweight in ounces of water
   - Week 2: Boost stomach acid with 1 tbsp. apple cider vinegar at meals
   - Week 3: Add in a daily probiotic and prebiotic
   - Week 4: Eat 2-3 different colors (veggies) each meal
   - Week 5: Sip herbal tea before bed and/or drink 1 cup meat or bone broth daily.

Phase 3 (Weeks 6+): Reintroduction & Maintenance Phase

Your Phase 3 Reintroduction & Maintenance Phase is ALL ABOUT experimenting with Mindful & Intuitive Eating.

During Week 6 and beyond you will have full liberty to experiment with many of the "20% foods" you avoided during your initial 28 days, as a testing ground for asking yourself: **How does food make me feel?**

Here's how:

1. Choose the food(s) you want to "test" for re-incorporating
2. Eat ONE* of the foods three days in a row
3. Note how you feel in a food log or journal (Bloating? Low energy? Brain fog? Skin breakouts, etc.)
4. Option to continue experimenting with other foods

*Only choose ONE new food at a time to reintroduce so you are really able to decipher what you need.

> **Gut Kickstart Tip: Eat in Abundance**
>
> During the Experiment phase, it's also encouraged that you continue to press toward a "LEAST RESTRICTIVE MINDSET"—eating as many real foods as possible (in abundance) according to the foods that sit best with you.
>
> Lastly, the Experiment phase is a time to customize your diet. Tweak or modify your supplement plan **and recognize trigger foods that don't sit well with you.** Instead of looking to GAPS, or AIP, SCD, low-FODMAP, Paleo or Vegan, Experimenting challenges you to look to YOU and do YOU. For instance, you may find white rice sits well with you, sweet potatoes make you bloat. Broccoli is great, but Brussels sprouts or kale are not your gut's best friend. Occasionally a little chocolate or homemade coconut ice cream never hurt and you don't have to be anti-sweets. You get the picture. Instead of any one diet, you do the YOU diet. After all, the word "diet" means "way of life" anyways.

Above All: Remember: 80/20

Before I set you loose, remember ABOVE all that the Gut Kickstart is meant to be sustainable (not a game of perfection). If you "mess up" or eat a food "not on plan" or forget to take a supplement one day, don't sweat it! 80/20, 80/20, 80/20—80% of the time, eating real whole foods, 20% of the time, let life happen. One last time, the BIGGEST question to continually ask yourself throughout the Reset: How do I feel? Let your gut feelings be your guide.

Is Healing REALLY Possible?!

Hippocrates said it best: "Healing is a matter of time, but it is also a matter of opportunity."

Thousands of people have implemented the tools and tricks from the 28 Day Gut Kickstart over the years only to discover that they didn't know how good they could feel, until they felt good! That said, for many, gut healing does not happen overnight. It is more of a marathon—not a sprint—especially considering how long you may have struggled with "gut issues" in the first place.

Your Resources section in the back of this book is full of tons of supporting Gut Kickstart Hacks and additions to add to any specific imbalances you may be experiencing—such as constipation, bloating, IBS and SIBO. However, remember the biggest game changers of them all: addressing stress and loving your gut from the inside out.

Hone in on the simple things—good food, clean water, good sleep, daily movement, daily breath, healing gut support, AND gut love (from your heart and soul), and you'll be unstoppable.

The remainder of this book includes tools and resources to help you put your plan into action.

Gut Kickstart Resources

1. The Gut Kickstart Rules — 296
2. 5 Daily Gut Love Habits Checklist — 297
3. Daily Journal Template — 299
4. Complete Gut Kickstart Food List — 304
5. Meal & Snack Ideas — 314
6. Experiment Phase 101 — 319
7. Intuitive & Mindful Eating — 321
8. The Psychology of Eating — 328
9. How to Conquer Your Cravings — 333
10. How Healthy is Your Poop? — 338
11. Gut Love Hacks: Additional Supplement & Lifestyle Supports to Add In — 338
12. Cheat Sheet Protocols: Constipation, Bloating, IBS, Allergies & Everything in Between! — 356
    - Next Level Hacks — 356
        - Abdominal Cramping — 356
        - Allergies — 358
        - Cold & Flu — 359
        - Dysbiosis/Fungal Overgrowth — 364
        - General Bloating & Constipation — 366
        - GERD — 372
        - IBS — 374
        - Leaky Gut — 377
        - Liver/Gallbladder-greasy stools — 381
        - Nutrient Deficiencies — 384
        - SIBO — 386
        - Skin Breakouts — 389
13. Detox 101 — 392
14. FAQ's — 403

The Gut Kickstart "Rules"

The "rules" of the 28 Day Gut Kickstart are a little different than most diet or clean eating programs out there.

Rule 1: Connect with Your Body

Continually check in with your body: "How do I feel?" Use your Intuitive & Mindful Eating Food Log to connect to how food makes you feel and also think!

Rule 2: Listen to & Eat for Your Body

There's no one-size-fits-all approach to "healthy eating." Toss out your beliefs about what is "healthy" and "unhealthy." Eat and implement gut healing practices and foods which work best for your body. For instance, nuts may be a healthy food, but may not be healthy for your gut (right now). White rice or fermented sourdough bread may be a grain, but when you reintroduce new foods, it actually may work just fine for you! Most important: **nutrients and foods should make you feel good.**

Rule 3: Conquer Your Cravings

We often crave foods we are intolerant to (thanks to our gut bacteria). Recognize when your gut bacteria may be crying out and continue to support and love your gut.

Rule 4: Be Patient with the Process

Time, consistency, listening and self-compassion pays off. Keep your eyes forward, while also not forgetting where you're coming from. Your gut "issues" didn't happen overnight, and it can take some time to "get out of it."

Rule 5: Keep an 80/20 Mindset

No perfection. A little dirt never hurt (in fact, it may be really good for you).

5 Daily Gut Love Habits Checklist

1. Hydrate:

Drink half of your bodyweight in ounces of water each day, beginning with 12-16 oz. warm lemon water first thing in the morning

Bonus 1: Drink your water in a stainless steel water bottle and opt for clean filtered water.
Bonus 2: Limit coffee to one 8-oz. cup each day
Bonus 3: Start the day off with 8-12 oz. fresh celery juice at least 20-30 minutes before eating.

2. Boost Stomach Acid:

Consume 1 tbsp. Apple Cider Vinegar in water 1-3 times per day

Hack: Add a teaspoon of pure maple syrup to Apple Cider Vinegar if you cannot stomach it.
Optional: Take an HCL Capsule or Tablet* https://llax.metagenics.com/spectrazyme-metagest-formerly-metagest if you cannot tolerate Apple Cider Vinegar

*not recommended if pregnant or taking PPI medications

Bonus: Take 1-2 digestive enzymes with meals, pause 1-2 minutes before meals to chew your food really well for maximized digestion.

3. Gut Kickstart Bugs:

Take a Soil-Based Probiotic + Prebiotic
Dose: 1 Probiotic in the morning and 1 in the evening; 1 Prebiotic Powder serving in the evening on an empty stomach

Bonus: Eat 1-2 condiment-sized servings of fermented foods and a prebiotic food each day.

4. Taste the Rainbow:

Eat 2-3 Colors with Meals & 2 Servings of Greens Daily

Bonus: Cook, steam, saute, dice, puree and peel veggies to optimize digestion. Raw veggies are more difficult to digest. Add 1-2 tbsp. healthy fats (coconut oil, olive oil, ghee, olives, etc.) with meals to assist in digestion.

5. Soothe:

Sip Herbal Tea in the evening.

Bonus: Candle down. Shut off screens 1-2 hours before bed. Read, connect, reflect on your 3 gratitudes.

Daily Journal Template

Here's a sample daily log journal you can keep throughout your Gut Kickstart—especially during the first couple of weeks and your Reintroduction Phase at the end to assess how certain foods, supplements and lifestyle factors make you feel.

Morning Log

Good morning sunshine!

_____

_____

_____

Gut Kickstart Affirmation

"This is my body. I love and accept it just as I am."

_____

_____

_____

Get Your Mind Right

I don't have to do it all. My top 3 priorities for today are…

1. _____

2. _____

3. _____

MY DAILY SCHEDULE

MORNING

_____
_____
_____
_____
_____

MID-DAY

_____
_____
_____
_____
_____

EVENING

_____
_____
_____
_____
_____

The 28 Day Gut Kickstart

MINDFUL FOOD LOG

Listen to your gut...

....
....
....

MEAL TIME

BREAKFAST ....

HUNGER **(BEFORE MEAL)** | FULLNESS **(AFTER MEAL)**

GASSY | BLOATED | CONSTIPATED | FATIGUE/ENERGY DIP | HEADACHE | SUGAR-RUSH
ENERGIZED | ANXIOUS | BORED | WORRIED
HOW I FELT

COMMENTS ....

LUNCH ....

HUNGER **(BEFORE MEAL)** | FULLNESS **(AFTER MEAL)**
HOW I FELT

COMMENTS ....

DINNER ....

HUNGER **(BEFORE MEAL)** | FULLNESS **(AFTER MEAL)**
HOW I FELT

COMMENTS ....

SNACKS ....

COMMENTS ....

WATER INTAKE

▯ ▯ ▯ ▯ ▯ ▯ ▯ ▯

PROBIOTIC: **Y | N**   FERMENTED FOOD: **Y | N** | Kefir | Yogurt | Sauerkraut | Fermented Veggies | Kvass | Kimchi   **Y | N**

Dr. Lauryn Lax

PROBIOTIC: Y | N   **FERMENTED FOOD:** Y | N   Green-Tipped Banana/ Plantain | Cooked & Cooled Potatoes/Squash | Onions, Garlic | Jerusalem Artichoke | Leeks   Y | N

SLEEP LAST NIGHT

HOURS ....

QUALITY
....
BROKEN | POOR | WELL-RESTED | NOTHING-SPECIAL | I COULD HAVE SLEPT MORE

MOVEMENT

....
WHAT I DID TODAY
....

THOUGHTS & FEELINGS ABOUT WORKOUT

Hard to Pass | Easy Peasy | Funky | Too Much | Small Amounts Several Times
ELIMINATION ....
                 TIMES   TIMES   EXPERIENCE

Sausage Like, But Lumpy | Sausage with Cracks | Sausage Snake, Smooth & Soft | Pellets, like nuts or pebbles | Soft Blobs | Thin Ribbons | Mushy & Fluffy | Loose & Watery | Smelly/Foul | Greasy
....
SHAPE & TYPE

Dark Brown | Light Brown | Gray | Greenish | Black   *SEE BRISTOL STOOL CHART
....
COLOR
....

CANDLE DOWN STRESS

TODAY I WAS STRESSED ABOUT
....
....

STRESS BUSTER TO USE
....
....

302

THREE COOL THINGS THAT HAPPENED/ GRATITUDES

1. ....
2. ....
3. ....

NOTES & THOUGHTS

Complete Gut Kickstart Food List

28-Day Gut Kickstart Food List

Consider these 28 days as a refreshing reset for you to be the one who decides what does and does not agree with your gut.

28-Day Gut Kickstart Foods

Nourish (Foods to Eat in Abundance)

PROTEINS

Note: Opt for organic, pasture-raised, and grass-fed meats as much as possible

- Additive-Free Protein Powder (Collagen, Beef Isolate, Cold-Processed Grass-fed Whey)
- Bacon/Turkey Bacon (nitrate-free, organic)
- Chicken (breast, thighs, whole, legs)
- Goat
- Grass-fed Meats (Beef & Grass-fed Bison/Buffalo; if you find you get constipated or upset stomach easily, limit)
- Hen
- Lamb
- Liver
- Meat Broth/Soup
- Organ Meats (heart, liver, tongue)
- Sausage (homemade, organic meat)
- Turkey/Ground Turkey
- Wild-Caught Fish & Seafood
- Wild-game Meats & Fowl (alligator, boar, pheasant, rabbit, venison, etc.)

HEALTHY FATS

- Avocado (1 small, 1/2 Medium, 1/3 Large=serving)
- Avocado Oil
- Bacon (organic, nitrate-free, pastured)
- Beef Tallow

The 28 Day Gut Kickstart

Coconut Butter
Coconut Flakes Unsweetened
Coconut Milk (additive-free; organic caned best)
Coconut Oil
Coconut Yogurt
Duck Fat
Egg Yolks (pasture raised, organic)
Extra Virgin Olive Oil
Fatty Cold Water Fish (Salmon, Sardines, Cod, Halibut, Tuna, Mackeral, etc.)
Fatty Cuts of Meat (grass-fed, organic, pasture raised)
Flax Oil
Ghee
Goat's Milk Butter
Grass-fed Butter
Grass-Fed Dairy* (Yogurt, Cream; No sugar, no additives, full-fat, plain; Limit amounts)
Grass-fed Goat's Milk
Lard, Non-hydrogenated
Mayonnaise (Avoid brands with canola oil or sugar)
Olives
Palm Oil, Red Palm Oil
Palm Shortening (for baking)
Pumpkin Seed oil

SEEDS

Moderation, 1 serving or less/day (1 serving=¼ cup or 1-2 tbsp. Sunflower seedbutter)

Chia
Hemp
Flaxseed
Pumpkin Seed
Sesame seeds
Sunflower SeedButter/Seed Butters
Sunflower seeds

NON-STARCHY VEGGIES

Leafy Greens

Arugula
Baby Greens
Basil
Beet Greens
Bok Choy
Butterhead Lettuce
Cabbage
Chard

Chinese Cabbage
Collards
Dandelion
Endive
Kale
Kelp
Lettuce
Mesclun
Mustard

Parsley
Power Greens
Romaine
Seaweed
Spinach
Sweet Potato Leaves
Swiss Chard
Turnip Greens
Watercress

Other Non-Starchy Veggies

Artichoke
Asparagus
Bean Sprouts
Bell Peppers
Broccoli
Brussels Sprouts
Capers
Cauliflower
Celery
Cucumber
Fennel
Garlic
Grape Leaves
Green Beans
Hearts of Palm
Horseradish
Kohirabi

Leeks
Mushrooms
Okra
Onions
Parsley
Pickles
Radicchio
Radish
Rhubarb
Sea Vegetables
Shallots
Snow Peas
Spaghetti Squash
Tomatoes, raw
Water Chestnut
Yellow Squash
Zucchini

STARCHES & TUBERS

Acorn Squash
Arrowroot Starch
Beets
Butternut Squash
Carrots
Cassava
Chayote
Coconut Flour
Delicata Squash
Jicama
Kabocha Squash
Parboiled Jasmine Rice (cooked and cooled, keep to 1-3 servings/week)
Parsnips
Plantain
Potatoes (red, Yukon, gold, purple, new, etc.)
Pumpkin
Rutabaga
Sweet potatoes (Jewel, Garnet, Jersey, Purple and Japanese—so many flavors!)
Taro
Turnip
Yam
Yuka

FRUITS

Acai Berry
Apple
Apricot
Banana
Blueberries
Blackberries
Boysenberries
Cranberries
Cantaloupe
Cherry
Coconut
Date
Elderberry
Fig
Goji Berry
Grapes
Grapefruit
Guava
Kiwi
Mango
Nectarine
Oranges
Lemon
Lime
Melons
Papaya
Peach
Pear
Persimmon
Plums

Pineapples
Passion fruit
Pomegranate
Pumpkin
Plum
Raisin

Raspberry
Starfruit
Strawberry
Tangerine
Tangelo
Watermelon

"DAIRY"

Goat's Kefir/Yogurt or Coconut Kefir/Yogurt
Non-Dairy, Unsweetened Goats Milk & Coconut Milk (additive & carrageenan-free)

PROBIOTIC FERMENTED FOODS

*eat in medicinal servings

Fermented/Pickled Veggies
Fermented Condiments (Mustard, Ketchup, Relish, Horseradish, Salsas, etc.)
Kefir (Water, Coconut)
Kimchi
Kombucha (low sugar like Health Ade brand—only 2 grams of sugar, or make your own)

Kvass (Beet Kvass)
Miso & Natto (fermented varieties, no-additives)
Sauerkraut
Tempeh
Yogurt (Coconut Yogurt; full-fat grass-fed dairy with "live and active cultures only)

PREBIOTIC FOODS

Apples
Asparagus (al dente)
Banana (Green-tipped)
Cabbage
Chicory

Cooked & Cooled Sweet Potatoes/Potatoes
Cooked & Cooled Tubers (Parsnips, Winter Squash, Carrots)

Dandelion greens
Eggplant
Endive
Fennel
Garlic
Raw Honey
Jerusalem artichokes
Jicama
Kefir
Leeks

Onions
Plantains (Greenish)
Radicchio/Radishes
Mushrooms (reishi, shiitake and maitake)
Potato Starch or Plantain Starch
Seaweed/Algae (Beta-glucan, or β-glucan—a soluble fiber)

BONUS: BEST GUT LOVING FOODS

Bone Broth
Beets/Beet Greens
Apple Cider Vinegar
Gut-soothing teas including chamomile, papaya, fennel and ginger tea
Dark Leafy Greens
Dandelion Root
Peppermint/Mint
Garlic
Ginger
Parsley
Cinnamon
Turmeric
Fresh Melons (Watermelon, Cantaloupe, Honeydew; eaten alone)

Lemon
Pineapple
Coconut
Wild-caught fish and seafood including tuna, sardines, salmon and even sea vegetables
Fresh organic vegetables
Sustainably Raised Meat
Organ Meats (liver, heart, tongue)
Healthy fats that are easy to digest, including coconut oil, avocado and ghee

SPICES & HERBS

Unlimited natural herbs and spices (except for nightshades)

Sea Salt
Basil
Bay Leaves
Black Pepper
Celery Seed
Chamomile
Chives
Cilantro
Cinnamon
Cloves
Coriander
Cumin
Dill
Garlic
Ginger
Horseradish
Kelp Granules
Onion Powder
Oregano
Mace
Majoram
Mustard Seed
Nutmeg
Parsley
Peppermint/Mint
Rosemary
Sage
Saffron
Salt (sea salt)
Tarragon
Thyme
Turmeric
Vanilla Bean
Any other **non-nightshade** natural herb or spice

SWEETENERS

Applesauce (unsweetened)
Banana
Coconut Butter
Cacao
Cinnamon
Dark Chocolate (moderation, 80-100%)
Fruits
Pure Maple Syrup (moderation)
Stevia (100% pure raw green leaf stevia, moderation)
Vanilla Extract
No other added sweeteners for 28 days (honey, molasses, splenda, etc.)

MISC & PANTRY STAPLES

Arrowroot Flour
Cassava/Tapioca*
(*Constipating for some

Coconut Aminos
Coconut Flour

Lifestyle "Nourishment"

- 7-9 hours of sleep each night
- Movement 3-5 days per week, with 2 rest/active rest days
- Clean, filtered Water
- Sunshine & Fresh air (30-60 minutes minimum)
- De-screen 2-3 hours before bed

Not Right Now: Top Gut Irritating Foods to Remove for Your kickstart:

Alcohol
Beans
Coffee (limit to 1 cup organic or none/day)
Corn
Chocolate
Dairy (except for grass-fed, full-fat sources, like grass-fed butter or ghee, or raw milk, Goat's Milk Kefir or Yogurt)
Dried Fruit
Egg Whites (Pastured Egg Yolks ok)
Limit restaurant meals
Nuts or Nut flours or Nut butters or Nut Milks (Sunbutter ok)

Nightshade Vegetables (white potatoes, tomatoes, peppers, okra, eggplant)
Nightshade Spices (paprika, cayenne pepper, capsicum, chili powder)
Sugar & artificial sweeteners (including honey, maple syrup, stevia)
Pork
Processed and packaged foods (*including* "gluten-free" packaged foods or "paleo" chips, bars, crackers; exceptions: coconut flour, arrowroot starch, cassava/tapioca)

Grains (oats, rice, pasta, breads)
Red Meats (limited to 3-4 times per week is recommended)

Soy (Tofu, Tofurky, Edamame, unless vegetarian/vegan and fermented source)

Vegetarian/Vegan Options & Exceptions:

Complete proteins are only found in whole-sourced proteins (meats, fish, poultry, eggs, etc.). If you absolutely do not eat meat as your protein source then a modified vegetarian/vegan approach to your Gut Kickstart Plan is as follows:

Additive-Free Protein Powder (Collagen, Gelatin, Pea, Hemp)
Eggs, Pastured
Fermented Tofu
Grass-fed Whole Fat Yogurt and Cheese
Raw Soaked Nuts & Seeds (1/4 cup serving)

Soaked Beans, Peas & Chickpeas
Soaked Quinoa
Spirulina
Tempeh, additive free, fermented
Wild Caught Fish

Your 28-Day Gut Kickstart is fairly simple—if it didn't grow on the land, swim in the sea or roam the earth, then it's not part of the Reset. The point of your kickstart Weeks are to "clean" any dirt off your windshield that MAY be dirty, so when the windshield is clean, you can actually see the specs of dirt that do or do not agree with your gut system.

Gut-Inflammatory Foods (Not Recommended at All)

- Any foods that upset your stomach
- Added sugar
- Additives
- Artificial sweeteners (aspartame, sucralose, acesulfame, saccarin, xylitol, sorbitol)

- Beans (canned, non-soaked)
- Candy
- Canola oil
- Cakes, pastries and other baked conventional goods and sweets
- Carrageen (found in some non-dairy milks)
- Cereal and Instant Oatmeal
- Coffee
- Coffee Creamers with additives and artificial sweeteners
- Condiments (with added sugar, high sodium)
- Conventional dairy
- Conventional eggs and meats
- Conventional, processed & refined wheat and grains (breads, crackers, pastas, granola bars, etc.)
- Corn
- Diet drinks
- Diet foods/bars/products
- Diet Butters/Spreads (like Smart Balance, Parkay, etc.)
- Frozen dinners with additives
- "Gluten-free" Products (made with LOTS of additives)
- High-fructose Corn Syrup
- Hydrogenated Oils (soybean, cornoil, safflower, peanut, cottonseed, canola, sunflower, ricebran oils)
- Ingredients with names you can't pronounce!
- Poor-quality coffee (Instant coffee; non-organic roasts; there are tons of toxins in coffee beans)
- MSG (packaged foods, frozen dinners, Chinese food)
- Nitrates in deli meats, sausages, hot dogs, bacon
- Pasta Sauces (with added sugars and chemicals)
- Peanuts
- Peanut butter and nut-butters with added sugar
- Protein Bars & Powders with artificial ingredients and chemical additives
- Salad dressings

- Soft drinks and fruit juices
- Soy
- Sports supplements with artificial sweeteners and additives
- Whey (with additives)
- Wheat (especially for the first 30-90 days, allow the gut to heal and digest optimally since wheat is one of the top food allergens)

Meal & Snack Ideas

GUT LOVE MEAL IDEAS

Breakfasts

28 Day Gut Kickstart
1. Turkey or Chicken Sausage + 1/2 Avocado + Pan-Fried Greens
2. Gut-Love Smoothie
3. Butter Bones: 12-16 oz. Bone Broth + 1 Tbsp. Grass-Fed Butter or MCT Oil + 1 Serving Collagen Powder
4. Salmon + Roasted Asparagus wrapped in Organic Bacon
5. Ground Turkey/Chicken + Butternut Squash + Greens + 1 Tbsp. Ghee

Experiment Phase
1. 2-3 Egg Omelet + Turkey Bacon + Spinach + Mushrooms + 1/2 Avocado
2. Ground Pork Herb Sausage + Fried Plantains + Greens
3. Steel-Cut Gluten Free Oats + Peaches + Cinnamon + Sunbutter + Additive-Free Protein Powder
4. Grass-fed Greek Yogurt + Frozen Berries + Collagen

5. Leftover Grass-Fed Bison + Greens + Butternut Squash + in 1 tbsp. Coconut Oil

Lunches

28 Day Gut Kickstart
1. Leafy Greens + Chicken or Fish + Sweet Potatoes + Oil & Vinegar + Avocado
2. Turkey Burger Patties in Lettuce Wrap with Mustard + Roasted Carrot Fries + Gut Love Ranch Dressing
3. Turkey on Coconut Flour Bread/Wrap + Avocado Oil Mayo + Sprouts + Lettuce + Crispy Brussels Sprouts Bites
4. Canned Wild Salmon + Roasted Veggies + Coconut Butter (1-2 tbsp)
5. Roasted Chicken + Roasted Veggies + Paleo Honey Mustard

Experiment Phase
1. Turkey/Ham on Sourdough Bread + Lettuce & Tomato + Avocado Oil Mayo + Cucumbers
2. Tuna Salad Collard Green Wrap + Sweet Potato "Chips" (Jackson's Honest)
3. Roasted Chicken + Goat Cheese + Greens + Tomatoes + Olives + Paleo Greek Dressing
4. Salmon + Quinoa + Greens + Oil & Vinegar
5. Grass-fed Burger Sliders with Lettuce & Tomato + Crispy Brussels Sprouts + Avocado

Dinners

28 Day Gut Kickstart
1. Baked Lemon Cod + Japanese Sweet Potato + Greens in 1 tbsp. Coconut Oil

2. Ground Turkey Tacos in Lettuce Wraps or Coconut Flour Tortillas + Guacamole + Summer Squash + Sauerkraut
3. "Creamy" (Avocado Oil Mayo Sauce) Spaghetti Squash with Roasted Chicken & Kale
4. Shredded Chicken BBQ (nightshade free sauce) + Roasted Carrot Fries + Avocado Slaw
5. Grilled Wild-Caught Salmon + Roasted Veggies in Olive Oil

Experiment Phase
1. Bison Steak + Mashed Cauliflower + Pan-fried Greens
2. Bean-less Chili with Greens & Ground Turkey + Coconut Flour Bread Cornbread with 1 tbsp. Ghee
3. Spaghetti Squash with Grass-fed Beef Meatballs
4. Pastured Pork Tenderloin + Small Sweet Potato + Greens in 1 tbsp. Coconut Oil
5. Herb Roasted Chicken + Jasmine Rice + Greens in 1 tbsp. Grass-fed Butter

GUT LOVE SNACK IDEAS

Snacks are optional. Incorporate one optional Gut-Loving Snack, dependent on your hunger-fullness levels. Eat to nourish your body and if you want a snack, check-in: Am I hungry or craving? Ensure you eat plenty of protein, fat and veggies at your regular meal times to help stave off hunger between meals.

Choose One:

- Cold Pressed Green Juice (green veggies + lemon)
- Bone Broth
- Piece of Fruit, Melon or Berries (1-2 Servings/Day; Best eaten alone or mixed in smoothie or easy-to-digest foods, such as a simple salad, coconut yogurt/yogurt in the morning or with 1 Tbsp. Coconut Butter, Sunbutter or Nut Butter - Experiment Phase only)

- Goat's Milk Kefir/Yogurt or Coconut Kefir (8 oz.)/Yogurt
- 1-3 oz. Protein (Leftover or Turkey/Ham Roll-ups, Canned Wild Salmon or Nitrate-free Jerky)
- Veggies + Healthy Fat (Guacamole + Paleo Ranch + Avocado Oil Mayo + Sunbutter, etc.)
- Healthy Fat: 1/2 Avocado, 1-2 Tablespoons Coconut Butter, Handful Olives, Coconut Flakes, Handful Seeds
- Beef Isolate or Collagen Protein Powder in Coconut Milk or Water
- Plantain Chips or Crackers with Guacamole or Dip (paleo ranch, bean free hummus, etc.)

GUT LOVE DESSERT IDEAS:

- Kefir (optional: frozen berries)
- Coconut Yogurt or Ice Cream (Homemade)
- Gut Love Chia Pudding
- Lemon Macaroons
- Cinnamon Baked Apple Slices
- Gut Love Cookie
- 80-100% Dark Chocolate Square

Basic Gut Love Supplements

During your first 28-Days, we are taking a "minimalist" approach—aiming to get the majority of your gut supports from food itself with a few additional supplement boosters. Here's your list:

Supplement List

- Soil Based Probiotic
- Prebiotic Fiber (like Partially Hydrolyzed Guar Gum)
- Digestive Enzymes (use as needed)
- Gut Healing Foods:
    - Apple Cider Vinegar or HCL Tablet (If not pregnant or taking PPIs)
    - Fermented & Prebiotic Foods
    - Bone Broth (optional)

Here's how to take them:

Pre-Breakfast
12-16 oz. warm lemon water
1 Probiotic

Breakfast
1-2 Digestive Enzymes
Apple Cider Vinegar (1 tbsp in water) or HCL Tablet with Betaine & Pepsin (600-700 mg)

Lunch
1-2 Digestive Enzymes
Apple Cider Vinegar (1 tbsp in water) or HCL Tablet with Betaine & Pepsin (600-700 mg)

Dinner
1-2 Digestive Enzymes

Apple Cider Vinegar (1 tbsp in water) or HCL Tablet with Betaine & Pepsin (600-700 mg)

Before Bed
Prebiotic 1-2 tsp in 8 oz water or tea
Probiotic
Herbal Tea

*Consume 1 condiment sized serving of a probiotic food and prebiotic food each day

Experiment Phase 101

After your 28-Day Gut Kickstart comes to a close, we aren't leaving you hanging just yet.

Weeks 6+ of your Gut Loving Program is where the fun begins: Hacking what it is your body truly does and does not agree with (right now).

During the Experiment Phase, you will get free choice to decide what foods you want to experiment with that you may not have incorporated during your kickstart (such as nuts, eggs, soaked grains, grass-fed dairy, chocolate, etc.).

Also use this time to conduct a "Re-Assessment" of any lab tests you originally ran approximately 30-90 days later.

How to Reintroduce Foods
I encourage you reintroduce foods one thing at a time, in three day increments, while noting how you feel around meals in your food log. Frequent consumption of processed, sugar-filled or refined foods is still not encouraged. Aim for real foods as much as possible, incorporating those "gray" gut-irritating foods at your discretion.

For example, you may choose to incorporate eggs back into your diet first.

During the Experiment phase, you'd include eggs three days in a row back into your diet and assess how you feel, before moving on to the next food you'd like to incorporate. In total, you will get through five experiments to finish out your program, but the ball is in your court if you'd like to continue experimenting beyond your 28-day journey.

The point of the Experiment phase is to equip you with the confidence, guidance and encouragement to trust your body (and go with your gut) so you can go on living your life post-program—recognizing your body wants to work for you (not against you).

By no means will your Gut Kickstart solve all your gut problems, but it will help you get a baseline upon which to build and customize your own gut-healing protocol, as additional foods are tolerated.

(Real) Food Examples for Experimenting:
- Pastured Pork
- Grass-fed Red Meat (more liberally than during the 28-Day Reset)
- Egg yolks and eggs
- Grass-fed Whole-Fat Dairy
- Nightshade Vegetables (white potatoes, tomatoes, eggplant, okra, peppers)
- FODMAPS (you initially suspected were causing you belly issues like apples, onions, or coconut)
- Nightshade Spices (paprika, cayenne pepper, capsicum, chili powder)
- Wine or Alcohol
- Quality organic coffee
- Nut-based Crackers

- Sourdough Bread
- 80-100% Dark Chocolate
- Corn on the Cob
- Fermented Tofu
- Hummus
- Black Beans
- Plantain Chips
- Soaked grains (quinoa, rice, steel-cut gluten free oats, etc.)
- Home-popped Popcorn

Ultimately, continue to think: **Eat with the least restrictive, abundance mindset and ask yourself: How do I feel?**

Intuitive & Mindful Eating

Chances are, if you're reading this book you already know you have some "gut problems" or digestive issues," however if you do have those gut problems, you may not be 100% aware of the blind spots keeping you stuck there.

Certainly there *could be* an underlying pathogen (like SIBO, Candida or yeast, parasites, or low stomach acid), but there may also be *every day* triggers and stressors perpetuating your gut health, unbeknownst to you.

This is where developing an Intuitive Eating & Mindful Eating practice come into play.

What is Intuitive & Mindful eating? I'm glad you asked!

Mindful & Intuitive Eating 101

"Mindful eating" and "intuitive eating" are often used interchangeably.

However, although they share *some* similarities, they are also very different.

- Intuitive Eating = Listening to your body and eating accordingly to its physical needs and cues.
- Mindful Eating = Eating with *intention* and *attention* to your body, mood and food.

Unlike intuitive eating's Emphasis on your body's **physical** cues, Mindful Eating tends to involve more **mental** engagement with your body, your schedule and daily needs.

What Intuitive Eating IS

- **Intuitive Eating varies from person to person.** Because our tastes, bodies, activities, emotions, and spiritual paths are different, what our bodies require in terms of nourishment also differs.
- **Intuitive Eating is cyclical.** Weekly, monthly, and annual cycles, even life cycles, change our body's need for, and responses to, food.
- **Intuitive Eating is imperfect.** Intuitive eating does not mean we'll always choose absolutely "healthy" or "pristine" foods. We won't always feel as if we've had a "perfect" balance.
- **Intuitive Eating does not mean we'll always choose absolutely "healthy" or "pristine" foods.** We won't always feel as if we've had a "perfect" balance.
- **Intuitive Eating is rhythmic** We feel pleasantly full (but not stuffed) after a meal and pleasantly hungry (but not starving) before the next.
- **Intuitive Eating includes a wide variety of foods.** Meats, fats, fruits and vegetables, and even starches play a role in normal intuitive eating. You don't restrict your body from the foods it was intended to thrive upon. And the exact balance and variety of foods must be individualized.

- **Intuitive Eating is free of obsession.** It acknowledges that our compulsions are due to biochemical or emotional reasons and any over- or under-eating is a clue to begin looking further as an opportunity for learning.
- **Intuitive Eating is nourishing to the body and spirit. It feels good.** Good food in the right amounts and at the right times excites the senses. It provides tactile and taste sensations as we eat, and a pleasurable "full" feeling afterward. When we finish a meal, we feel comforted and renewed - physically, emotionally, and even spiritually.
- **Intuitive Eating is is an essential component of self-care.** What better way to nurture ourselves than with the foods we need and enjoy in the amounts we require?

What Intuitive Eating is IS NOT

- Eating because your bored
- Eating past your level of fullness regularly
- Counting calories or measuring your food
- Fearing what food may do to your body
- Eating out of emotion or compulsion
- Planning and scripting out your meals for the day
- Keeping food rules for yourself
- Feeling guilty when you eat something that's not "healthy"
- Eating the same thing every day
- Trying to be perfect with your food

What Mindful Eating IS

- **Mindful Eating** is eating lunch on your work break at noon—even though you're not super hungry yet—because you know you won't get another break until 6 p.m.
- **Mindful Eating** is sometimes eating even if you don't feel like it—because you know your body needs enough fuel

- **Mindful Eating** is trying the chocolate chip cookie your mom made especially for you when you travel home—even though you don't eat a ton of sweets regularly.
- **Mindful Eating** is cooking turkey sausage instead of eggs and bacon in the morning, because you've come to realize eggs make your belly feel nauseous.
- **Mindful Eating** is stashing a couple snacks in your purse to have on hand for later if or when hunger strikes.

What Mindful Eating is NOT

- Worrying over the half of a cupcake you just ate
- Neeeeeeding something sweet to make a meal complete
- Carefully scripting or planning out your meals—what you'll put in your mouth (or what you won't)
- Pre-planning what you'll order at the restaurant next week or calling the hotel to see if they can accommodate your sweet potatoes and turkey burgers you bring on vacation
- Eating out of boredom
- Closet eating
- "Earning" your food
- Eating because your have to or it's part of your checklist
- Restricting all day, then loading up at night

Intuitive & Mindful Eating in Practice: 10 Tips

Want some other ways to begin incorporating *more intuitiveness and mindfulness* into your Gut Kickstart Program? **Try some of these simple "gut loving" techniques to connect more to your gut and food:**

1. Breathe
Before diving into your plate, sit down and practice conscious breathing a few times to bring your body and mind together. After meals do the same thing. Take your time—you don't go swimming right after you eat, so don't race around or dive back into work the second you're finished, either.

2. Be Present.
Practice the art of being present with both yourself and for the food in front of you. Taste your food. Smell your food. Appreciate the food you're eating (if you don't do this, your body won't either). Focus. Turn off the TV, iPhone and laptop. Put away the newspapers, magazines, mail or homework. Experience the textures of your food. Soak up the fellowship and company around you.

3. Slow Down.
Savor small bites and chew your food thoroughly. Eat slowly—even if that means putting your fork down between bites. Allot 20-30 minutes for a quality meal.

4. Eat with Your Gut.
Serve a modest portion to start on a smallish-medium sized plate. If you are truly still hungry after you've finished your portion, then considered seconds.

5. Eat Freshly Cooked, In-Season Foods.
If your food isn't fresh, you won't feel as fresh after eating it. Skip the heat-and-serve frozen stuff, bags, packages and boxes as much as possible in favor of real foods cooked.

6. Shun Food Fads.
Keeping up with the latest on what to eat, how, or when, can be a challenge. After all, what works for a million other people may

still not be right for you, as each of us is a unique being. Loving your gut is the art of whole living—not a fad. Eating real foods that nourish and energize *your body* has been around since the beginning of time.

7. Uncover the Roots.
Recognizing common patterns of GI discomfort—not just foods—can help you connect more to your gut, and uncover the roots of improper digestion. Some may include:

- Eating late in the evening when the body is ready for rest and not prepared for the heavy work of digestion. (Eat a lighter, well-cooked meal at least two to three hours before bed, and try to be in bed around 10:00 p.m. or before).
- Eating raw veggies or heavy meats which are difficult to digest.
- Having weak digestion due to an imbalance or to stress.
- Poor hydration. When the body is not hydrated, it cannot remove impurities from the lymph system properly. Blood production and flow may be negatively affected, possibly inhibiting our body's ability to carry and maintain oxygen and nutrients.

8. Eat for Your Soul
Gut Kickstart nourishment goes beyond physical wellness to well-being in mind, spirit, emotions and senses. The food we eat nourishes our mind and emotions, not just our body. Cooking and eating in a harmonious atmosphere turns food into nectar. A pleasant, tidy, cheerful environment and the nurturing company of friends or family also makes mealtimes more nourishing and absorbable. The same goes for the mindset with which we approach our meals. If we *believe* our food will cause us gas, bloating or discomfort (prior to eating it), what do you think will happen? More than likely: Indigestion. If we believe our mom's

homemade spaghetti is enjoyable and nourishing for our body *and* soul (even though we don't always eat grains), we are more apt to digest what we eat.

9. Experiment with What Your Eat
Eat the same dishes several times a week? Does your grocery list have the same items on it each time? Variety is the spice of life. Eating the same old dry chicken and broccoli strips all the fun and joy (i.e. deliciousness) from the meal. And when Vitamin P goes down (Vitamin Pleasure) so does our digestive system, mood and inspiration for nourishing ourselves with nutrient-dense foods. Get in the kitchen and whip out a recipe (or experiment) with making your own concoction.

10. Drink Warm Water & Ginger Tea. It's good for banishing bloating, sluggishness and upping energy (hydration). Ice cold water actually stalls digestion and can make you feel worse—i.e. disconnected from your body.

Bonus: Keep a Log!
Throughout your 28-Day Gut Kickstart, you're encouraged to keep a Mindful Food Log or journal—especially during the first two weeks—to help you begin to develop the skills of Intuitive & Mindful Eating. This log will include:

- What you ate
- How you felt around meals (Physically, mentally, emotionally, gut symptoms)
- Record your level of hunger and fullness (on a scale of 1 to 10, with 1=famished and 10=stuffed) around meals

Note: Calorie counting apps, like MyFitnessPal are NOT recommended. The purpose of logging your food is not to count calories, macros or obsess over what you eat. Quite the opposite! The goal is to wean you off overthinking food at all *and* feeling amazing—equipping you to become 100% in-check with your body—how it feels, your hunger and fullness around meals, enjoyment of the foods you eat, and freedom to trust your body and your own gut feelings (instead of labels, rules or noisy fads).

The Psychology of Eating 101

Beyond hunger and fullness, and how you feel physically, your **mental relationship** with food also influences your **connection** to your **body**.

Oftentimes with gut "issues," we recognize we don't feel 100 percent in our gut or body, but we continue to do the same things and eat the same things because change is hard or our mind plays tricks on us—keeping us stuck.

In addition, digestive issues can bring up a variety of emotions and beliefs around food, such as fear (fear of foods causing us harm or discomfort) or strict rules (orthorexia, obsession with healthy eating or perfectionism around diets).

The psychology of eating—the reason why we eat what we eat—goes beyond the act of eating itself or simply following the rules t a certain diet prescribes.

Check in with the deeper reasons that influence what we eat, how we eat, and how we feel:

Food as Identity.
Are you paleo? Vegan? Vegetarian? AIP? GAPS? The diets we follow sometimes become part of our identity—governing our food choices above how our body (or gut) feels when we eat some of the foods on that diet. In addition, culture, religion, age, gender and ethnicity can influence our food identities and can serve as both roadblocks to our own healing (i.e. eating foods that may

not agree with us) as well as accelerators (i.e. finding peace and positive connotations with our food).

Food as Judgment.
How do you judge yourself based on your eating habits? How do you judge others? Our judgments about food and diet can hold us back or propel us forward. For instance, do you feel self-conscious about eating an autoimmune-based protocol or refraining from drinking—even if it makes you feel great? Or do you judge others who eat their processed foods and feel like you earn your gold start if you stick to your strict SCD lifestyle? Judgment around food can increase stress over food, consequently decreasing digestion.

Food as Self-Sabotage.
Fear of succeeding with a change we want to make or fear of failing if we make a lifestyle or nutrition change can keep us stuck in our same patterns, routines and ruts of eating foods that don't make us feel great.

Food as Emotion.
Eating when you're bored, sad, or even celebratory can trump listening to your body—even if the peanut butter or milkshake tastes good.

Food as Fear.
Do you have certain beliefs about food which govern your choices about what you eat? Such as, "Carbs make you fat," or "Too much fat will store on your thighs." When we eat out of fear (rules) for our body, rather than love, we may miss out on some key nutrients or provoke a stress response around meal times.

Not Trusting Our Body.

Lack of trust in our body's desire for health and healing causes more stress. Similar to eating out of fear and not love, when we think our body (and digestion) is working against us, we lack peace around meal times. This is common, especially amongst those who have struggled with constipation, bloating, IBS, GERD, a chronic disease or some other GI issue repetitively for a long time. They grow used to their body always feeling "at war" with itself, and consequently, develop a lack of trust (and sometimes even hate) for their own health and body. Your gut senses this.

Reflection: Understanding Your Food Philosophy

Similar to your Gut Timeline you created, what is your Food Philosophy—and how has it changed over the years?

Your food philosophy are your specific beliefs about what you eat and why you eat it—your personal food psychology. Take 5-10 minutes to whip out a pen and paper and jot down what your current food philosophy is, as well as how it's changed since your childhood.

What would you want your ideal food philosophy to look like?

Healthy, gut-loving you?

Good vs. Bad Foods

There's no such thing as "good" and "bad" foods."

It's a body-positive statement you've probably *heard* before, right up there with "everything in moderation"…but is it **really** true (especially since it's advised you "cut out" some foods for 28 days)?

After all, we *know a* McDonald's cheeseburger and French fries have a completely different nutrient profile than say a chicken breast and sweet potato.

And we *know* what the better option is when we compare a Snickers bar to an apple.

So is there **really** such a thing as "no good or bad foods" or "everything in moderation" (when the truth seems sooooo obvious)?

The answer?

You decide.

Allow me to explain this truth….

"Is it good?" or "Is it bad?" is not a distinctive "yes," or a "no."

Instead it is 100 percent customized answer to you—depending on your heart, head, experiences and personal health status.

The views, attitudes and relationships we have with our bodies, our food and ourselves are FAR more important than the nutrition labels, or stereotypes, of any food we put into our body.

For example:
An Egg McMuffin is not "good" for me (especially if I eat a lot of processed foods regularly or if I am looking for the most optimal, energizing nourishment).

However, to an extent, an Egg McMuffin was actually "good" for me in my recovery from my eating disorder when I was forced to eat it in treatment, because it made me braver (beyond food). As much as I hated eating an Egg McMuffin, I lived to tell about it, and it helped me realize that what does not kill me, makes me stronger.

Although I don't believe eating them weekly was the best option for my gut health, in part, eating an Egg McMuffin in treatment allowed me to also realize:

a.) I can go on vacations or social party with food—out of my control—and go with the flow, and

b.) Eating an Egg McMuffin also allowed me to realize how much better I feel when I am nourishing my body with real whole foods—and inspired me to explore and integrate my "food as medicine," philosophy in the later years (for the first time, embrace real, whole fresh foods as life-giving nutrition to my body, mind and soul).

See the difference?
True, certain foods *do* have more nutrients than others, and there is no denying that REAL food—the simple foods like animal proteins, vegetables, fruits and healthy fats (like avocados, coconut oil, olive oil, fatty fish and nuts/seeds) are foods your body thrives upon.

BUT…when I label foods as "good" or "bad," I give food a greater life and control of its own and set myself up for the diet mentality.

Eat in "Abundance"
This is a methodology I practice today which helps bring clarity to the dilemma at hand—and I am going to teach you how to do the same.

It means eating with the "least restrictive as possible" viewpoint.

When you begin the art of intuitive eating (listening to your own body), you begin to recognize how certain foods truly make you feel/don't feel and what foods are good for your own gut health, mind health and energy.

"Eating in abundance" means maintaining an "abundant" mindset—"What *CAN I eat?*" *in*stead of a restrictive mindset (*What do I have to eliminate?*).

Instead of saying, "I CAN'T have that," or "That's BAD for me"… We say things like:

"What CAN I have?" and "How am I nourishing my body?"

The answer may very well become clearer.

The Bottom Line
"Good" and "bad" foods don't exist.

Yes, more nutrient-dense foods DO exist.
Less nutrient-dense and nourishing foods DO exist.
And "good" and "bad" mentalities DO exist.

But if you….

- Aim to eat more nutrient-dense foods in abundance
- Tune in to how certain foods do and don't nourish your body (how you feel, breakouts, gut health, etc.)
- Go on strike from unnecessary rules
- Embrace opportunities to challenge old diet mentalities
- And realize there is NO such thing as "perfection" or "perfect eating"

Then freedom is yours for the taking!

How to Conquer Your Cravings

Did you know our gut bugs often crave foods we are *intolerant* to?

If you have some bacterial overgrowth or imbalanced gut flora with more "bad" bacteria than good, your "bad bacteria" feast off of foods you are intolerant to and will signal to your brain for you to "feed" them with the very foods that you crave (but don't make you feel good).

Why does our brain hijack our body and make us all confused around what we really want or what our body really needs?!

Is *listening* to a craving "intuitive eating?" Or are cravings bad and should you try to deny them at all cost?

Aye! Aye! Aye! THE STRUGGLE IS REAL!

Cravings 101

Cravings are a mixed bag, and they can actually be *both* "intuitive" and "**mental**" or *emotional*.

Here's the difference:

Intuitive Craving: A cellular hunger, deficiency or body signal cueing you "I am missing something here." (i.e. "I need some iron from red meat," "I need some magnesium from chocolate," "I need some healthy fats for energy—I am dipping.")

vs.

Mental or Emotional: Your mindset or emotions are driving the show because your mind and heart tell you that you'll *feel better* (or less bored, less sad, less uncomfortable, more satisfied) if you just have X ("If you just have coffee, you'll have more energy." "If you just have something sweet, your tastebuds will be satisfied.).

Cravings are NOT a bad thing.

The only time they become "not a good thing" is when they control you.

The difference in a **healthy craving** vs. a "craving gone wrong" is when those cravings **take over**. When they hijack your feelings, thoughts and emotions—and those feelings, thoughts and emotions *don't go away* until that craving is satisfied. And, often, even after the craving is satisfied, you are still left thinking about *that food, or that craving.*

On the other hand, an **intuitive** craving for chocolate (magnesium) for instance may strike around your period. You may not understand why you want chocolate, but by listening to your intuitive craving, you eat some chocolate…and you're satisfied (and not necessarily thinking about the next time you can eat some chocolate).

Like riding a wave, you let the waves of cravings come and go. You listen to them. But then you're good.

You're not left thinking, planning or salivating for the next time you "can have it." You're not feeling guilty for "giving in" to it. You don't overthink how you can "make up for it" in your workout.

You're satisfied, until the next wave comes, when maybe your body tugs at you:

"I want some refreshing watermelon!"
"You know what—nuts really don't sound good today, I felt pretty bloated when I at them."
"A piece of pizza sounds delicious."

No judgment. No more thought than just—food is food, and you let your body lead in nourishing you, eat to satisfaction, and build the majority of your nourishment upon real foods, letting "life happen" occasionally when that pizza does sound good (versus letting your mind and emotions dictate what you do and don't eat).

The bottom line: Cravings are NOT a bad thing.

When you do get a craving, check in: Does my body want it, or do I "neeeeeed" it, and is this a healthy (mindset) for me? The answers will help you decipher how to proceed.

SO WHAT DO I DO STILL IF I AM CRAVING SOMETHING?!

Good question. The answer is up to you decide. Often, constantly craving the same things happens because:

a.) We are intolerant to the foods we crave (and our gut bugs feast off them)

b.) We are missing other essential nutrients in our diet (or not eating enough during the day). This causes our blood sugar to drop and our body cue us to reach for our craving.

c.) We keep doing the same habits and rituals around the foods we crave and eat (like watching TV every night and needing popcorn every night when we do that activity).

d.) We have unaddressed emotions we are not talking about or in check with (loneliness, poor self-esteem, bored in our lives, etc.)

Check in with yourself—do any of those fit for you?

CONQUERING CRAVINGS

The best way to conquer a craving?

Two things:

#1 Do Something Different
If we don't do something different in our lives—whatever it is—nothing (cravings included) will change.

Mix it up.

Instead of sitting on the couch to eat your usual bag of popcorn and wine, sit on a yoga ball to watch TV or stretch on the floor—chances are this new trigger will make you at least think before the same habit takes over.

With sweets, instead of completely denying your craving, reach for a protein or fat-based snack and portion it out on a plate or away from the container.

Lastly, **think in the POSITIVE** (not the negative): "It's not bad to have a craving," "My cravings do not control me," or "I can nourish my body with an abundance of fresh foods."

(When we think in the affirmative—rather than the negative, we quit "wanting what we can't have" as badly).

#2 Eat in Balance

Focus on making sure your body is getting the energy it needs and you ARE eating *enough* by eating balanced meals throughout the day.

If your basic needs are NOT being met, then of course you're going to crave SOMETHING for energy and satisfaction—(and typically a quick source of energy and satisfaction, like sugar, coffee or a crunchy salty snack).

To **reset** your cravings:
Aim for three balanced meals per day.

For the average moderately active woman (lifestyle movement + 3-5 days of exercise during the week) this looks like at least:

- 5-6 oz. of protein (1-2 hand sizes)
- Veggies (half your plate, especially leafy greens)
- 1-2 healthy fat sources with each meal (coconut oil, coconut butter, ghee, grass-fed butter, 1/2 avocado, handful nuts or seeds, olive oil, olives, avocado oil)

Add in:
Half your bodyweight in ounces of water each day. **Plus**, 1-2 starchy veggies (sweet potatoes, beets, carrots, squashes, etc.)

and 1-2 fresh fruits per day (carbs are your friends) as well, and you're golden.

As for snacks, if you *do* need snacks throughout the day, great! Reach for a protein or fat as the base of your snacks to help stave off blood sugar drops.

It doesn't get much simpler than that.

#3 Check In
If a craving for a snack or sugar STILL strikes…Check in.

Cravings are NOT bad. A gut-check-in can point your towards whether it is a *want* (mental, emotional, low blood sugar, gut bug craving) or *legit* body need.

Respond accordingly.

How Healthy is Your Poop?

Check out the Bristol Stool Chart in Chapter 7A to see where you measure up.

Gut Kickstart Hacks: Additional Supplement & Lifestyle Supports to Add In

Here's an overview of some general helpful supplements that many with digestive distress may benefit from.

Note: Start out slowly with the supplements and gradually increase your doses as tolerated. Recommendations are intended for a general audience and are not to be considered the best treatment for your individual needs. For a customized approach, it is best to connect with a practitioner who can help guide you in lab testing and implementing appropriate treatment for test findings.

Basic Nutrients

Cod Liver Oil.
What's It For? Constipation, Bloating, Skin Breakouts, Allergies/Low Immunity, Brain Fog, Malabsorption
Fatty acids aid in digestion serve as a lubricant for helping food ease down the digestive tract. Deficiencies in fat acids have been linked to various intestinal disorders and diseases—particularly in those with a history of low-fat diets or an intake of inflammatory fats (i.e. vegetable oils, fried and greasy foods) are more at risk for digestive distress. Fatty acids also help all the vitamins and minerals you eat in your food "stick," since fat aids in absorption in the first place. Fats in our food sources are found in saturated fats (grass-fed butter, ghee, coconut oil, organic meats and eggs), monounsaturated fats (olives, olive oil, avocados, flax seed), omega-3's (fatty fish like salmon, tuna and sardines, walnuts, pastured eggs, grass-fed beef/bison) and polyunsaturated fats (seeds, flax, nut butter) and we require a blend of all fatty acids for optimal health (inside and out). Of the fats we consume, Omega-3 fatty acids are *essential* because our bodies don't actually make them on our own (our body can synthesize other fats if it must). They are also, arguably the toughest for many to get in our western diets since many folks don't eat fish often. That said, try a supplemental Omega-3, preferably from an extra virgin cod liver oil for maximum absorption (cod liver oil contains Vitamin A and Vitamin D, which aids in absorption of the fatty acid).

Get it: Add 1 teaspoon of cod liver oil to your supplement routine; Continue to aim to have 1-2 healthy fats through your food sources as well at meals.

Vitamin B12
What's It For? Constipation, Low Stomach Acid, IBS, No Appetite, Nausea
Vitamin B12 deficiency is thought to be one of the leading nutrient deficiencies in the world, with 40 percent of Americans having low levels. Vitamin B12 is responsible for your central nervous system and metabolic function, thus when we are low, our metabolism and nervous system of our digestive system suffers. Deficiency is associated with low stomach acid, constipation, poor appetite, nausea, and diarrhea. In addition, **other B-Vitamins play a role in digestion as well:**

B1 (thiamine): Helps your body change the carbohydrates in your diet into energy for your cells and to regulate appetite. **B 3 (niacin):** Important for many digestive tract functions including the breakdown of carbohydrates, fats, and alcohol.
B6 (pyridoxine: Helps process the protein you eat
Biotin: Helps your digestive system produce cholesterol and process proteins, carbohydrates, and fatty acids.

Get It: Vitamin B Complex + Folate or Methylfolate Complex (folate ensures the proper uptake of Vitamin B-12). The foods with the most B vitamins include organic liver and organ meats, as well as organic meats and wild-caught seafood (salmon, clams, sardines, crabs and mussels).

Vitamin D
What's It For? Low energy, Malabsorption, Fatty Acid Deficiency, Calcium Deficiency and Vitamin/Mineral Deficiencies, Constipation, Low Thyroid
Also known as the "sunshine" vitamin, **Vitamin D is the only vitamin we can get from another source other than food** (a minimum of 15 minutes of sunlight each day), in addition to some foods (cold-water fatty fish or shellfish) and supplements. Vitamin D is critical for health. It enhances calcium absorption

in your gut and maintains adequate calcium and phosphate levels in your blood, ensuring your bones stay strong. Vitamin D is also an anti-inflammatory vitamin. Many studies have shown a link between low Vitamin D and inflammatory bowel disease since Vitamin D may help the immune system to reduce levels of inflammatory proteins that get overproduced. Unfortunately, Vitamin D deficiency is extremely common, with studies finding upwards of as many as 70 percent of Americans deficient. The ideal range of 25(OH)D Vitamin D is 35-60 ng/mL for whites, and a little bit lower (30-60 ng/mL) for non-whites.

Get It: 15-60 minutes of sunshine daily + 1 lb. wild caught fatty fish each week/pastured egg yolks + 1 tsp./day of Extra Virgin Cod Liver Oil supplement (there are various cofactors which are required for the absorption of certain nutrients that are present in food that are not present in synthetic Vitamin D supplements, thus food and cod liver oil are ideal before Vitamin D alone); if levels on your bloodwork are:

Below 15: Supplement with 10,000 IU/d D3 each day
Between 15-25: Add in 5,000 IU/d D3 each day
Between 26-35 with PTH (parathyroid hormone levels) >30: Add 1 tsp. cod liver oil + dietary changes and sun exposure
Between 26-35 with PTH (parathyroid hormone levels) <30 and >35: No supplementation is necessary

Magnesium
What's It For? Constipation
Magnesium is crucial for regulating cell cycles and growth, as well as apoptosis, or cell death. Without enough of it, our digestive process slows down and many people experience constipation, bloating or lack of appetite with magnesium deficiency. Since a positive side effect of magnesium is the relaxation of muscles and organs—your digestive system included—without enough of it, your digestive organs are not relaxed to allow food

to move through. Blood work can help determine your deficiency status and if magnesium levels are below 2.0 mg/dL you could more than likely benefit from some magnesium.

Get It: Magnesium Glycinate Supplement (200-500 mg per day for adult males and 200-400 mg per day for adult females, aim for upper end if you are deficient). In addition, the ideal food sources with magnesium include clams, green chard, spinach, beet greens, kelp, basil (fresh), kale, chives, coconut water, okra and arugula.

Additional Digestive Support Aids

Antimicrobials or "Botanicals"
What's It For? Bacterial Overgrowth & SIBO, Constipation, Bloating, Parasites, Gut Bugs
Antimicrobials are herbs and herbal supplements often used along with probiotics and targeted nutrients to help reestablish a healthy gut microbiome.

Plants have been used as primary medicine for centuries and antimicrobial supplements consist of various blends of herbs in one capsule, such as oil of oregano, thyme, berberine extracts, and wormwood, which work against gut imbalances like antibiotics do for illnesses—"attacking" the disease, inflammation and overgrowth of any bacterial overgrowth in your gut.

Antimicrobials are like "natural" antibiotics that make your body more resilient and irradiate any gut bugs attempting to throw your healthy bacteria out of balance. Although antimicrobials are commonly used to specifically treat SIBO (small intestinal bacterial overgrowth), they can also be beneficial if you experience bloating, constipation, IBS, digestive upset, colic and gas pain, and other signs of inflammation regularly.

Get It: Natural antimicrobial supplements are herbal in nature. Rifaximin is an antibiotic that has "antimicrobial" properties specifically for treating SIBO and IBS-D; See Supplement Recommendations in your Resources section for specific brands.

Antifungals
What's It For? Bacterial Overgrowth, Parasites, Fungi, Dysbiosis
Antifungals are a *type* of antimicrobial, specifically used to treat fungal infections. Whereas other antimicrobial supplements target more than just fungi (like bacterial overgrowth and foreign invaders in the gut), antifungals are specifically used when fungal infections or yeast overgrowth are found in stool cultures.

Get It: Antifungal supplements are typically a blend of herbs, such as: thyme, turmeric, yerba mansa, burdock, black walnut, echinacea, paracress and myrrh. One of my top recommended antifungals is Lauricidin, which contains the antifungal Monolaurin—a 12-carbon long fatty acid, derived from coconut oil, which has antibacterial and antiviral properties to kill off gut bugs. It also is a natural component of breast milk for babies—the perfect food—making it a powerhouse for rebuilding the immunity of your gut. As a supplement, Monolaurin is a "non-toxic antibiotic" which does not appear to have an adverse effect on gut healthy bacteria. See Resources section for additional recommendations.

Anti-Biofilm Enzymes
What's It For? Bacterial Overgrowth, Parasites, Fungi, Dysbiosis, Leaky Gut
Biofilms are microorganisms (bacteria) which adhere to a surface and have two sides—some are "good" (they make your gut strong to fight off disease, infection, antibiotics and toxins, as well as keep our digestive tract working) and some are "bad" (strong enough to cause tooth decay, gum disease, sinusitis, ear

infections, brain disease, cancer, heart disease, keep wounds from healing, keep bladder infections recurring, etc.). They naturally line the digestive tract, especially the lower intestines. Healthy biofilms contain many different species of bacteria working together to benefit humans. However, in the case of stressors like bacterial overgrowth, parasitic infection and dysbiosis, we have less healthy biofilms, leaving us susceptible to all sorts of inflammation and disease.-

Get It: Anti-Biofilm enzymes help release agents to fight off the bad biofilms in our gut if dysbiosis or fungal overgrowth/infection is present. Take apart from other supplements, between meals to ensure you don't kill off any other helpful enzymes or botanicals (herbs, antimicrobials) you may be taking.

Prokinetics
What's It For? Constipation, SIBO, Bacterial Overgrowth, IBS-C
Prokinetics are substances that increase gastrointestinal *motility* by stimulating the strength or the frequency of contractions in the small intestine. These can be herbs or combinations of herbs or drugs.
Get It: MotilPro or Iberogast are available over-the-counter. Herbs include Ginger, Chinese zhi zi (fructus aurantii), and Chinese jin yin hua (flos lonicerae).

Ox Bile
What's It For? Improves fat digestion and absorption and supports your liver and gallbladder in bile production (especially if you've had your gallbladder removed)
Bile acids are naturally produced in your liver and then flow into your gallbladder where they are stored and concentrated to assist your digestion in breaking down fats we eat. However, if you have a sluggish gallbladder/liver from inflammation, toxic overload or gallbladder surgery, your body will struggle to break down fat. Ox Bile to the rescue! .

Get It: Beta Plus by Biotics

Glutamine
What's It For? Intestinal Wall Healing, Leaky Gut, Stomach Ulcers
Glutamine is an amino acid which has been linked to intestinal permeability restoration (helping heal the gut lining). In fact, your GI tract is the greatest user of glutamine in the body because it provides the primary fuel for the nutrient-absorbing cells that line the walls of the small intestine. It is found in protein-rich foods like Bone Broth, Grass-fed Beef/Bison, Grass-fed Raw Dairy, Wild-Caught Fish, Turkey, Spirulina and some veggies (asparagus, broccoli, and cabbage). However, when you have leaky gut, the body's tissues need more glutamine than the amount consumed in the diet and internal production.
Get It: Supplemental L-Glutamine Powders (2-5 g/day), add 1 scoop to water

Zinc
What's It For? Leaky Gut, Frequent Constipation or Bloating
Zinc aids your body in over 300 enzyme functions—including digestion, appetite and energy production (from your foods). Low zinc is connected with low zonulin (the key protein that holds together your gut wall and tight junctions) and **consequently leaky gut** (Skrovanek et al, 2014). Essentially, without enough zinc, you don't have enough zonulin and you're more apt for leaky gut. Zinc, like cortisol, has a diurnal rhythm, so zinc levels will vary through the day, which makes accurate testing and lab work difficult (levels will change in a given day). If you do run blood work, you want levels between 64-126 (for zinc) and 81-157 (for copper—the great zinc equalizer nutrient). At home, the best way to test for overall zinc deficiency and your need for supplementation is the zinc taste test. All you need is a bottle of aqueous supplemental zinc (like Biotic Aqueous Zinc)

and 30 seconds. Take a spoonful or two swig of the zinc and swish it around in your mouth for 30 seconds, note your signs and symptoms.

Zinc taste test measures:
- Very deficient: No specific taste sensation, tastes like plain water. This indicates a major deficiency of zinc.
- Semi-Deficient: No immediate taste is noticed within the first 10-15 seconds of the test, then a 'dry' or 'metallic' taste is experienced.
- Slightly Deficient: An immediate slight taste is noted, which increases over the next 10 seconds.
- Adequate/Optimal: An immediate, strong and unpleasant taste is experienced. This indicates no zinc deficiency exists.

Get It: If your zinc is low in this taste test or your blood work, add a 15 mg/Zinc supplement to your daily routine until your taste test improves. (Note: Those who follow a vegetarian or vegan diet may require up to 50 percent more zinc than omnivores since they do not consume animal meats). Foods with high zinc are organ meats, wild-caught fish/shellfish and organic pastured meats.

Natural Herbs & Oils

In addition to supplements you find on a shelf, here is a quick hit list of some of the top medicinal therapeutic herbs and natural agents which boost gut health:

Activated Charcoal	Curcumin
Aloe Vera	Berberine
Castor Oil	Essential Oils
Chamomile	Frankincense
Cinnamon	Garlic
Coconut Oil	Ginger

Licorice
Marshmallow Root
Oil of Oregano (Emulsified)
Peppermint
Turmeric
Slippery Elm

Lifestyle Interventions

Aside from supplements, herbs and oils, there are also *tons* of alternative gut-healing therapies and treatments out there which may compliment your custom Gut Kickstart Protocol.

Some popular alternative gut-healing interventions include:

Acupuncture
Coffee Enemas
Colonics
Deep Breathing
Juice cleanses and broth cleanses
Hot-cold therapy
Hypnosis
Iridology
Particular dietary interventions (GAPS, AIP, SCD, etc.)
Prayer
Psychotherapy
Meditation
Ozone Therapy
Saunas
Tai-Chi
Yoga

With so many options, it can feel a bit overwhelming knowing where to start.

For the purpose of this book and your program, we don't have the time to go into each one of these in-depth, and this is where your own experimentation may come into play. Some may work for you, others will not.

A large part to figuring out your gut-healing puzzle is to be the experiment. It doesn't hurt to try, and if you fall down and skin your knee, you can always get back up, having learned from it.

That said, above all, remember once more that while it can be easy to want to try EVERYTHING under the sun to "heal your gut," the **tried and true method (that you cannot go wrong with) is:** Keep it **simple**.

Don't discount the power of your basic gut healing protocol + lifestyle interventions + addressing stress, and this one game-changing intervention (you are going to get really good at).

(Move over coffee enemas and sauna therapy.)

Baseline Gut Health Maintenance: Lifestyle & Nutrition Recommendations

Stress is the #1 driver of all disease—including gut imbalances—so stress reduction is critical for improving symptoms. You cannot out-supplement a stressful lifestyle or poor diet. Here are some essential strategies.

Eat an Anti-Inflammatory Nutrient-Dense Diet.

- **Eat in Abundance:**
    ▷ Proteins—Grass-fed meats; pastured & organic poultry, eggs and pork; wild game; wild-caught fish
    ▷ Carbohydrates—Color-rich, nutrient-dense fresh vegetables, starchy tubers and roots, and fruits
    ▷ Healthy Fats—Plant and animal fats (coconut and coconut oil, olives and olive oil, ghee, grass-fed butter, lard, duck fat, pastured egg yolks and fatty cuts of organic meats, some raw nuts and seeds, avocado)
    ▷ Bonus Gut Healing Foods: Fermented foods, bone broth, fresh herbs and spices, apple cider vinegar

▷ LOTS of Fresh, Clean (filtered) Water
- **Limit or Avoid:**
  ▷ Industrial seed oils and hydrogenated fats (canola oil, grapeseed oil, vegetable oils)
  ▷ Sugar and artificial sweeteners (not just candy bars; often hidden in bottled smoothies, granola bars, cereals)
  ▷ Dairy (except kefir and plain, full-fat grass-fed yogurt for prebiotics as tolerated)
  ▷ Many "healthy" marketed packaged products: Instant oats, whole grains
  ▷ Most protein powders and bars
  ▷ Instant coffee, alcohol (limit to 4-6 drinks per week), sodas, sports drinks, juices
  ▷ Most grains and gluten*
  ▷ Corn
  ▷ Beans* and peanuts
  ▷ Soy
  ▷ Most processed gluten-free products (exceptions: avoid gums, reach for products with coconut flour, arrowroot and/or tapioca/cassava)
  ▷ Most packaged and processed foods
  ▷ MSG and other food additives and food colorings
  ▷ Limit SPICY foods (Sriracha, red pepper flakes, paprika, chili powder, peppers)
  ▷ In short: The modern day Western (Standard American) Diet.

Some people find they do ok with a little bit of white rice, grass-fed dairy, whole soaked beans, quinoa or gluten-free oats, but for an initial 30 days it's often best to take these out to then experiment with how they affect you. **The Bottom Line:** Eat real foods MOST of the time, with an 80/20 balance (perfection is impossible and should never be expected).

Practice Anti-Inflammatory Lifestyle Habits

This is where the REAL fun begins. Beyond putting good food into your mouth, the nutrients you put into your life also are huge game changers. Stress—no matter how many greens you eat—is constantly going to be the "elephant in the room," until addressed. Some examples to limit stress include:

- Sleep 7-9 hours each night
- Incorporate a variety of movement (strength, aerobic, mobility, power) 5-6 days per week or at the very least, daily lifestyle movement (cleaning, walking, moving—not sitting for hours on end)
- Replacing your tap water and plastic water bottles with clean filtered water and a stainless steel water bottle.
- Take time to play and pursue your passions and interests (overwork leads to burnout and that "gut feeling" of stress)
- Avoid stimulants in the afternoon/night (coffee, energy drinks)
- Soak up the sun and fresh air (humans need sunshine like a plant needs sunshine and water)
- Detox your home and beauty products in favor of more natural products
- Start your day off with a mindful morning routine (before stress and the rat race gets the best of you: Don't check your social media and email first thing, but read a mindset boosting devotional instead; stretch or move your body.
- Candle down in the evenings (avoid LED/artificial light at night to promote and maintain Circadian Rhythm function, which is aligned with digestive health)
- Practice Digestive Hygiene
- Chew your food real well
- Slow down and breathe before eating

- Eat undistracted (not working in front of a computer or watching a screen)
- Don't eat on the go
- Cook and home prepare the majority of your meals
- Eat fresh organic foods as much as possible
- Consume leftovers within 3-5 days max of prep
- Consume frozen meats within six months for ground meats and one year for muscle meats (throw out old)
- Address mental stress (talk about it)
- Connect to community and deep meaningful relationships
- Consider adding in a mindfulness practice (meditation, deep breathing, yoga, Tai Chi, prayer)

No, you do NOT have to do all of these things at once. Start with one which could be the most game-changing for you, and go from there. (Once you get the ball rolling, it's hard not to want to do more to feel even better and bring your body back to balance).

Rebuild a Healthy Gut Ecosystem

Add in three Baseline Gut Loving Supports, including:

- **Daily Probiotics & Probiotic Foods.** Healthy Gut Bacteria.
- **Daily Prebiotic & Prebiotic Foods.** Helps your probiotics "stick."
- **Apple Cider Vinegar.** Boost stomach acid naturally.
- **Digestive Enzymes**

Probiotics & Prebiotics

All long-term gut healing protocols should include both probiotics and prebiotics for optimal results. Probiotics and prebiotics are both essential to healing the gut.

Probiotics are healthy sources of bacteria which help to balance the health of gut bacteria in the gut, regulate immunity, and decrease gut inflammation.

NOTE: Probiotics are only maintainers of healthy gut bacteria in the gut. They do NOT increase the numbers of beneficial bacteria in the gut and do NOT colonize it with more species of healthy bacteria over time. That's because many species of probiotics that we take in supplements cannot "stick" in the gut, without prebiotics in conjunction.

Prebiotics are fibers found in supplements and foods which DO increase the beneficial bacteria over time because they provide food for those beneficial species of bacteria.

NOTE: It is sometimes necessary to avoid prebiotics early in the treatment process because in certain cases they can make conditions such as small intestinal bacterial overgrowth (SIBO), parasite infections, and fungal overgrowth worse, since bacteria are ALREADY overgrown in these conditions. Instead, treatment may focus on killing off bad gut bacteria first with antimicrobial herbs *then* adding in prebiotics.

Food Sources of Probiotics:
Coconut Yogurt
Fermented Veggies (carrots, zucchini, cucumbers, etc.)
Grass-fed Full Fat Plain Yogurt
Kefir
Kombucha
Relish (fermented)
Sauerkraut

Food Sources of Prebiotics:
Asparagus, al dente
Cooked & Cooled Sweet Potatoes, Potatoes, Carrots & Winter Squash (butternut, acorn, etc.)
Garlic
Green-tipped Bananas & Plantains (and plantain chips)

Jasmine White Rice, parboiled
Jerusalem Artichoke
Jicama
Onions
Mushrooms (reishi, shiitake and maitake)
Nutritional Yeast
Potato Starch or Plantain Starch
Seaweed/Algae (Beta-glucan, or β-glucan—a soluble fiber)
Soaked & Sprouted Beans (cooked and cooled)

Supplements:

Best probiotics for constipation:
Soil-based organisms
Seed Daily
Transient commensals
E. coli Nissle
Lactobacillus plantarum
Bifidobacteria infantis

Best probiotics for diarrhea/loose stools:
Soil-based organisms
Transient commensals
Saccharomyces boulardii
VSL#3
Elixa

Prebiotics:
Acacia
Unmodified potato starch
Glucomannan powder (pretty well tolerated, second best)
Partially Hydrolyzed Guar Gum (VERY well tolerated)
Psyllium husk powder
Modified Citrus Pectin

Digestive Enzymes

Optional Habit: Take 1-2 Digestive Enzymes with Meals.

What Are They? Digestive Enzymes are like a PAC-MANTM' for digestion—they help eat all the food and break it down along the path.

What to Take: Go to any nutrition shop or grocery store and you're sure to find dozens of digestive enzyme formulas to choose from. Like with any supplement, use caution. Just because the label says "digestive enzymes" does not mean it is a quality digestive enzyme or the right enzyme for you.

How Much? One to two capsules with your first few bites of food at your primary meals.

A couple rules of thumb when looking for the right enzyme for you:

1. **Aim For Quality**: Buying cheap supplements is a waste of money (you're almost never going to get the benefit you're looking for). When buying enzymes, don't look for the cheapest brand on the shelf and steer clear of conventional grocery stores and drug stores, as they carry poor quality product. Most quality brands will have more than one digestive enzyme listed (multi-strain), a strength amount listed (if strength is not listed, be wary) and an ingredient list (You do not want: soy, dairy, wheat, sugar, salt or any other funky additives).

2. **Get the Right Support:** Depending on the level of support you need (i.e. carbohydrate breakdown, fatty acid breakdown, protein breakdown), there are certain enzymes which can help you more than others. See the Resources for a Guide to Enzymes.

Basic Digestive Enzyme Guide:
Not all enzymes are created equal. Varying your enzymes up and stacking them can give your gut an extra boost of "gut love"—such as taking a pancreatic enzyme as your base, then a gluten-specific enzyme for the times you travel or eat out. Here's the scoop:

All Around Support
Pancreatic enzymes provide a booster for all sorts of foods and can be a solid choice if you don't notice one type of food in particular (fats, proteins, or carbs) is more difficult to digest than others. Pancreatic enzymes contain the "big three" enzymes: Protease, Amylase and Lipase, which should come into play once food hits the small intestine (the organ where the majority of digestion happens). Pancreatic enzymes are particularly helpful for those who have food allergies or sensitivities, since pancreatic enzymes are critical to proper protein digestion.

Gluten & Carbohydrate-Specific Enzyme Formulas
Some digestive enzymes are specifically made with the consumption of carbohydrates and gluten in mind. These are great to have on hand for those times you get "brain fog," experience bloating, or get a blood sugar dip after eating a carb-heavy meal. These are also great for eating out at restaurants when food may be cross-contaminated with gluten or if you suffer from SIBO (small intestinal bacterial overgrowth).

Fatty Acids-Liver/Gallbladder Enzyme
If you feel queasy after eating fats of any sort (fried or restaurant foods, healthy fats like red meat, butter or avocados), a liver/gallbladder enzyme support can help with easing the gallbladder's and liver's role in digestion. I recommend a mix which contains digestive and antioxidant enzymes, as well as vitamin C, taurine, and organic beet concentrate for special liver/gall-bladder support.

Next Level Hacks

Cheat Sheet Protocols: Constipation, Bloating, Allergies & Everything in Between!

Abdominal Cramping 356
Allergies 358
Cold & Flu 359
Dysbiosis & Fungal Overgrowth 364
General Bloating/Constipation 366
Gerd 372
Ibs 374
Leaky Gut 377
Liver/Gallbladder Dysfunction 381
Nutrient Deficiencies 384
Sibo 386
Skin Conditions 389

Abdominal Cramping

Chronic abdominal cramps are typically related to some other underlying issue such as SIBO, IBS, dysbiosis, food intolerances, zinc deficiency and/or leaky gut, gastritis, parasites, liver/biliary congestion, ileocecal valve disturbance or upper GI bleeding.

- **Assess for underlying pathogens in both upper and lower GI through testing and self assessment, including:**
    - ▷ Zinc Deficiency (taste test or blood work)
    - ▷ Urine Test for indican and sediment levels
    - ▷ Stool Analysis (parasite profile and comprehensive digestive analysis)

- ▷ Food Intolerance Testing
- ▷ SIBO Testing
- **If a pathogen is found, then address accordingly. In the meantime, "Immediate" Short-Term Relief for cramping includes:**
  - ▷ Find a position (such as on your hands and knees, downward dog or curled up) which helps alleviate some pain.
  - ▷ Swig 1 tbsp. of apple cider vinegar in 2-4 oz. of water
  - ▷ Consume some fermented food (sauerkraut, ginger kombucha—low sugar)
  - ▷ Drink warm herbal tea
  - ▷ Don't lie on your back directly after eating
  - ▷ Go on a walk
  - ▷ Chew on garlic
- **For upper intentional cramping, some additional helpful supplements include:**
  - ▷ HCL + Pepsin Tablet
  - ▷ Pancreatic Enzymes
  - ▷ Digestive Enzymes with Bromelain, cellulase, lipase and amylase
  - ▷ Beet juice, taurine, Vitamin C and pancrelipase support (Beta-TCP by Biotics)
  - ▷ Zinc-15 mg/day
- **For lower intentional cramping, some additional helpful supplements include:**
  - ▷ Probiotics and Prebiotics
  - ▷ Antifungal Herbs
  - ▷ Butyrate
  - ▷ Fiber
  - ▷ Micro Emulsified Oregano

Allergies

In addition to eating real food and your basic digestive protocols, combat allergies and low immunity with these methods:

- Double Up on Probiotics and/or Fermented Foods. A short term therapeutic dose.
- Avoid High-allergenic and Inflammatory Foods: Grains, nuts, legumes and peanuts, shellfish, sugar, coffee, artificial sweeteners and dairy.
- Add 1-2 tbsp. Apple Cider Vinegar to water and tea (3-6 times per day)
- Incorporate Pineapples for Bromelain (reduces swelling in nose and sinuses), plus leafy greens, wild-caught fish and organic meats, garlic, onion, ginger, cayenne and probiotic-rich foods (full-fat fermented yogurt/goats milk yogurt, kefir, sauerkraut, fermented veggies, etc.)
- **Supplement Savvy**—Some additional helpful aids to add to the mix:
  - **Add L-Glutamine Powder to** water. (Healing for intestinal lining)
  - **Liposomal Curcumin** keeps inflammation at bay. (1 dose)
  - Add **Spirulina** to your smoothie, tea or water; or take a capsule (to stop histamine release)
  - Support the immune system with **Mircro-Emulsified Oregano** http://llax.metagenics.com/mp/products/candibactin-ar and **Garlic** (natural or *supplemental*)
  - **Take Herbal Antihistamines.**
  - **Take "True Tonic" or Fire Cider (an apple cider vinegar concoction)** Sip 1-2 Tbsp. in the morning and at night. https://d-chi-kitchens.myshopify.com

- ▷ Food Intolerance Testing
- ▷ SIBO Testing
- **If a pathogen is found, then address accordingly. In the meantime, "Immediate" Short-Term Relief for cramping includes:**
  - ▷ Find a position (such as on your hands and knees, downward dog or curled up) which helps alleviate some pain.
  - ▷ Swig 1 tbsp. of apple cider vinegar in 2-4 oz. of water
  - ▷ Consume some fermented food (sauerkraut, ginger kombucha—low sugar)
  - ▷ Drink warm herbal tea
  - ▷ Don't lie on your back directly after eating
  - ▷ Go on a walk
  - ▷ Chew on garlic
- **For upper intentional cramping, some additional helpful supplements include:**
  - ▷ HCL + Pepsin Tablet
  - ▷ Pancreatic Enzymes
  - ▷ Digestive Enzymes with Bromelain, cellulase, lipase and amylase
  - ▷ Beet juice, taurine, Vitamin C and pancrelipase support (Beta-TCP by Biotics)
  - ▷ Zinc-15 mg/day
- **For lower intentional cramping, some additional helpful supplements include:**
  - ▷ Probiotics and Prebiotics
  - ▷ Antifungal Herbs
  - ▷ Butyrate
  - ▷ Fiber
  - ▷ Micro Emulsified Oregano

Allergies

In addition to eating real food and your basic digestive protocols, combat allergies and low immunity with these methods:

- Double Up on Probiotics and/or Fermented Foods. A short term therapeutic dose.
- Avoid High-allergenic and Inflammatory Foods: Grains, nuts, legumes and peanuts, shellfish, sugar, coffee, artificial sweeteners and dairy.
- Add 1-2 tbsp. Apple Cider Vinegar to water and tea (3-6 times per day)
- Incorporate Pineapples for Bromelain (reduces swelling in nose and sinuses), plus leafy greens, wild-caught fish and organic meats, garlic, onion, ginger, cayenne and probiotic-rich foods (full-fat fermented yogurt/goats milk yogurt, kefir, sauerkraut, fermented veggies, etc.)
- **Supplement Savvy**—Some additional helpful aids to add to the mix:
  - **Add L-Glutamine Powder to** water. (Healing for intestinal lining)
  - **Liposomal Curcumin** keeps inflammation at bay. (1 dose)
  - Add **Spirulina** to your smoothie, tea or water; or take a capsule (to stop histamine release)
  - Support the immune system with **Mircro-Emulsified Oregano** http://llax.metagenics.com/mp/products/candibactin-ar and **Garlic** (natural or *supplemental*)
  - **Take Herbal Antihistamines.**
  - **Take "True Tonic" or Fire Cider (an apple cider vinegar concoction)** Sip 1-2 Tbsp. in the morning and at night. https://d-chi-kitchens.myshopify.com

The 28 Day Gut Kickstart

- **Quercetin.** 1000 mg/day to stop the release of histamine.
- **Cod-Liver Oil** to boost immune fighting Vitamin A stores.
- **Zinc.** 30 mg/day for a short-term dose.
- Drink **Ginger, Dandelion-Root Tea** or other **Herbal Tea** at night (http://llax.metagenics.com/mp/products/glutagenics (Bonus: Add raw honey)
- Sip **Bone Broth** or Meat Broth

Cold & Flu

80% of your immune system is in your gut. Forget the Tylenol Cold & Flu, Campbell's Chicken Noodle Soup & sugary cough drops. **Boost immunity with these 15 Natural Cold Remedies to Heal Faster—No Medications Needed:**

Probiotics
Since more than 80% of your immune system is housed in our gut, what do you think happens when our gut bugs aren't happy? We are more prone to illness. Boost your gut with a double dose of **soil-based probiotics** when facing a cold, flu or allergy attack.

Apple Cider Vinegar
Similar to how probiotics boost healthy bacteria in your gut, Apple Cider Vinegar also boosts gut health by boosting stomach acid—essential for a proper functioning gut and digestion. Add a spoonful to 2-4 ounces of water and swig with your meals.

Oregano Oil
An essential oil that is considered to be antibacterial, antiparasitic, antiseptic, antiviral and immune stimulating. Like the fresh herb, Oregano Oil has very high amounts of antioxidants. It is

often used internally during illness, and externally for skin infections (including yeast), though it should be diluted with a dab of coconut oil before use. Buy as an essential oil http://amzn.to/2D-B99qS and dilute one drop with one drop coconut oil or extra virgin olive oil and take under the tongue. To get the full benefits of oregano oil, use a dosage of 50-100 mg oregano oil 4x per day.

Castor Oil
The "windex" of all things wellness, castor oil has the ability to "speed up" healing by increasing white blood cells and the count of T-11 cells (a type of special white blood cells that act like antibodies) produced within the body's lymphocytes that help kill viruses, fungi, bacteria and cancer cells. Rub the oil http://amzn.to/2zQ8mAk on pulse and sinus points, and the back of the neck.

Turmeric
A natural anti-inflammatory agent for calming the inflammatory response in the body. **Curcumin**, the active ingredient in turmeric, is antiviral and antifungal. Use a Liposomal Curcumin http://amzn.to/2DBZAYG for a supplement formula, or add turmeric spice to recipes, like Turmeric Tea https://autoimmunewellness.com/anti-inflammatory-turmeric-tea/, Turmeric Milk https://heartbeetkitchen.com/2015/recipes/seasonal/winter/soothing-turmeric-milk/, Anti-inflammatory Meatballs http://eathealthrive.ca/moroccan-sweet-potato-meatballs-aip-paleo-whole30/ or Turmeric Ginger Carrot Soup http://gourmandeinthekitchen.com/ginger-turmeric-spiced-carrot-soup-recipe/.

Garlic
Whole garlic contains a compound called alliin. When garlic is crushed or chewed, this compound turns into allicin, the main active ingredient in garlic which boosts the disease-fighting response of white blood cells in the body when they encounter viruses.

How to "take" it? Garlic can be crushed, chewed and/or cooked into food. Crush or slice garlic before you consume it to increase the allicin content, add to a spoonful of applesauce, or add into dishes at meals. Bonus: Try Wellness Formula. A power-packed multi-vitamin with a base of herbs, including garlic, in one place. http://amzn.to/2zQpoyf

Vitamin C
Ascorbic acid, or Vitamin C, has long been touted as an "immune booster." Add a little more to the diet through citrus, strawberries and spinach during illness, and short term supplementation via 1000 mg of Liposomal Vitamin C (Empirical Labs http://amzn.to/2CfDqzm, Seeking Health http://amzn.to/2BZSlK5). Liposomal formulas are more absorbable.

Elderberry
An essential oil and food linked to decreased cold and flu duration due to antibacterial and anti-infectious qualities. Use organic dried black elderberries (1 http://amzn.to/2CpYDU5, 2 http://amzn.to/2DB8Axo) to consume whole, or make a homemade syrup with this recipe:

Elderberry Cold "Medicine"
Ingredients:
2/3 cup dried black elderberries (about 3 ounces)
3.5 cups of water
2 Tbsp fresh or dried ginger root
1 tsp ground cinnamon
1/2 tsp clove powder
1 cup raw honey

Directions:
Pour water into medium saucepan. Add elderberries, ginger, cinnamon and cloves (do not add honey). Bring to a boil and then cover and reduce to a simmer for about 45-60 minutes until

liquid is reduced by almost half. Remove from heat and let cool enough to be handled. Mash berries using a spoon. Pour through a strainer into a glass jar or bowl. Discard elderberries and let liquid cool. Add one cup of honey and stir well.

Essential Oils
Natural healing agents to infuse into your home and air, like a natural vaporizer. Reach for peppermint, lemon, lavender, eucalyptus, cinnamon, clove and grapefruit.

Homemade "Cough Syrup"
Mix 2-3 tsp. raw honey with 1-2 ounces lemon juice. Dilute in water if needed.

Bone Broth
Move over Campbells, REAL bone broth is packed with antioxidants and gut-healing compounds to support all around immune boosting. Order it if you don't want to make, such as Osso Good Bones https://www.ossogoodbones.com, Fond Bone Broth http://www.fondbonebroth.com & BonaFide Provisions http://bonafideprovisions.com.

Water
The most life-giving and universal healing "supplement" of all. The body uses water, particularly during times of illness, to hydrate and flush toxins out of the body. Reach for a clean filtered source (on tap), and infuse with citrus (orange, lime, lemon, grapefruit) for an extra Vitamin C boost.

Green Juices
Get your greens (and antioxidants) to fight free radicals or make a green smoothie to ensure extra nutrients from an otherwise lost appetite. For juice, buy cold pressed greens https://drinkdailygreens.com/green-juices with no more than

one fruit, or just lemon/lime as the "sweetener." For green smoothies: Mix coconut milk or water with spinach, one fruit (choose: 1/2 green apple, frozen strawberries, orange slices or chunks of pineapple), cucumber, celery and parsley or cilantro and sip up!

Cold Busting Foods
This may seem like a no-brainer, but times of illness are particularly crucial for gut-loving and immune boosting foods including:

Citrus & Berries
Garlic
Onion
Ginger, peeled, raw or powder
Turmeric Spice
Cinnamon
Greens (raw and cooked)
Cruciferous Veggies (broccoli, cauliflower, Brussels sprouts)
Coconut Oil
Sustainable Proteins (pastured chicken, grass-fed meats)
Wild caught salmon
Bone broth
Natural Herbs (oregano, thyme, sage, rosemary)
Fermented foods
Prebiotic Foods (green-tipped plantains, bananas, cooked and cooled potatoes/sweet potatoes, cooked and cooled Jasmine white rice, artichokes, onions, leeks)

Rest
"Starve a cold" by giving the body ample time to heal during sleep and rest (when it recovers most).

Avoid

These may also seem like no-brainers, but while you're at "boosting your immune system, make sure these culprits are far away:

- **Sugar & refined grains:** These foods stress the adrenals (stress hormone production), feed yeast, and increase imbalanced gut bacteria.
- **Chemical additives:** GMO's, artificial sweeteners, food dyes, and other toxins stress the liver and the immune system.
- **Hydrogenated oils & fried foods:** Promote inflammation and decrease immunity and hormonal health. Nerves and brain function are also affected.
- **Repetitious eating:** The foods one becomes sensitive to are usually those eaten on a daily basis. A simple rotation diet minimizes stress to the immune system from hidden allergies. Try eliminating common allergens such as wheat and other grains, dairy, corn, soy, citrus fruits, chocolate, coffee, and soda.

Processed and packaged foods: These foods are devoid of real nutrition. Processed and packaged foods create nutritional deficiencies, diminishing one's health and vitality.

Dysbiosis & Fungal Overgrowth (Parasites)

There is a two-stage approach to restoring a healthy, balanced gut flora and ridding of any pathogens (fungus and parasites included).

Step 1: Get rid of or reduce pathological organisms. Use the same antimicrobial treatment as for SIBO for approximately 30 days. Additions may include:

Saccharomyces boulardii (healthy fungus)

Certain prescription medications, such as Alina or nitazoxanide may be prescribed for short term parasitic treatment

Step 2: Restore healthy gut bacteria (prebiotics & probiotics). Take soil and spore-forming probiotics in the morning, midday and evening, along with a serving of prebiotic fiber, like partially hydrolyzed guar gum, daily, AND plenty of prebiotic and probiotic foods (1-2 servings daily).

Supplement Savvy
Some helpful aids to add to the mix:

Start with 3-7 days of:

- **Digestive Enzymes** (1-2, taken with meals)
- **Emulsified Oregano Oil** (100-200 mg taken with meals)
- **Probiotic-Soil Based Formula** (start with 1 in morning for first 3 days, then add 1 at night)
- **Prebiotic Supplement** (1/2 tsp-1 tsp, away from meals)
- **Apple Cider Vinegar** (1 tbsp in 2-4 oz water) **or HCL Tablets** (1-2 with meals)

Then transition to:

- **Activated Charcoal** (mid-morning, 1 dose taken away from other supplements/food)
- **Anti-Biofilm Enzyme** (like Interfase Plus by Klaire Labs in mid-morning and mid-afternoon)
- **Anti-Fungal & Botanical Herbs** (1 dose in morning with breakfast and 1 dose night with dinner)
- **Monolaurin** (Lauricidin supplement, 3000mg, with each meal)
- **Ox Bile** (1 dose with each meal)
- **Probiotics-Soil Based Formula** (1 in morning, 1 midday and 1 at night)

- **Prebiotic Supplement** (continue to build up in 1/2 tsp doses every 3 days until a full dose is reached, away from meals with probiotic)

Notes:

- Ensure you're drinking water throughout the day
- Don't avoid carbs (anti-Candida diet is not recommended for most). Eat balanced while undergoing treatment, but avoid foods that flare symptoms.
- Optional: Rifaximin (alternative to antifungal and botanical herbs; prescription antibiotic for killing off overgrowth may be warranted if initial herbal protocol does not work well)

Severe Fungal Overgrowth Considerations:
If you have severe fungal overgrowth or imbalance, the following additional supplemental supports may be helpful:

Biotin (5 mg per day with meals)
Molybdenum (150-200 mg with meals)
Activated Charcoal (2-6 capsules/day, away from meals)
AFNG by Byron White (10-30 drops/day)

Dietary Considerations
Avoid "anti-candida" diets, since bacteria can thrive off ketones as well. Stick to your Gut Kickstart protocol

General Bloating, Gas & Constipation

Bloating, gas and constipation are common conundrums which stem from a lot of different underlying pathogens and stressors (SIBO, dysbiosis, food intolerances, etc.). Maybe you don't experience them ALL the time, but you experience them enough to be uncomfortable. The best thing you can do is first test and assess the main triggers of bloating and constipation. Also, keep a mindful food log to note any patterns or symptoms you notice flare up around certain foods, stressors or times of day.

In the meantime, for bloating and constipation relief, here is an arsenal of immediate and long-term bloating defenders: *Note: Some of these may sound like a broken record, but lifestyle measures will get you far.*

Prevention: General Bloating & Constipation

Probiotic. A probiotic is essentially a "gut-guard" helping your body manage inflammation in your gut, as well as kill off bad bacteria—like food fermenting in your gut.

Slow Down. Digestion MUST occur (optimally) in a parasympathetic state (i.e. relaxed). If your body is STRESSED while trying to digest, digestion is going to be that much harder. Slow down. Chew your food well. Breathe. Take breaks between bites.

Drink Water *Throughout* the Day. Water allows our juices (internally) to keep flowing and metabolic processes (including digestion) revving all day long. Kickstart your mornings—first thing before eating or drinking anything else—with 16 oz. of lemon water, and aim for a minimum amount of half your bodyweight in ounces of water each day. Note: *Avoid large amounts at meal times.*

Keep a Food Log. For 3-7 days, log what you eat plus what time you eat, your level of hunger and fullness, your total water intake throughout the day, as well as movement and sleep—this log is not to count calories or 'diet,' but to investigate. Before and after your meals, note how you feel (mentally, physically, emotionally, etc.).

Cut Out the Culprits. Dairy, gluten, sugar, and alcohol are common known gut irritants—but there are other foods which may equally affect you—like nuts, eggs, legumes (peanuts, beans), gluten-cross contaminating foods (potatoes, whole grains, rice, coffee, corn, soy, and chocolate) and some FODMAP foods.

Common FODMAPs include: artichoke, beans, apples, avocado, cauliflower, cabbage, coconut, processed meats, cashews, pears, cherries, onions, and of course, artificial sugars. Other common intolerances some people have are nightshade fruits and vegetables, including: potatoes, tomatoes, eggplant, Goji berries and black pepper.

You don't necessarily have to cut out everything. Use your food journal to help you problem solve.

Daily Nutritional Supports
- Drink half your bodyweight in ounces of clean, filtered (Start with your lemon water)
- Cook your greens and veggies (eat at least three servings per day)
- Incorporate healthy fats with every meal to lubricate your digestive tract
- Soak nuts, grains and seeds in water overnight prior to preparing
- Experiment with taking out dairy (or stick to full-fat organic plain versions only)
- Experiment with taking out coffee and fizzy drinks/carbonation
- Avoid large portions of meats and starches together in one setting
- Eat Fermented Foods 1-2x Per Day (sauerkraut, fermented yogurt, low-sugar kombucha)
- Incorporate beets a few times per week

Move your body. Get up and move throughout the day with lifestyle movement (i.e. short walks, a set of squats, pushups, yoga poses, etc.). Take intermittent breaks at work keep you from staying stuck in one position for too long (i.e. stuck at your desk). Moderate amounts of movement help prevent bowels from staying stuck. (Warning: Intense exercise—especially after meals can do the opposite and suppress digestion).

Take Your Time. Do you ignore the urge to go? If you don't go when you feel the urge, your constipation or bloating during the day can slowly worsen. Make time in your morning routine to sit down and try to go. If you strain while you go, invest in a Squatty Potty which supports the natural squatting position. You can also mimic this position by leaning back when you are sitting in the loo and pulling your knees towards your chest into a squat-like position.

In-The-Moment-Relief: Bloating

Assume the Position. Put a little yoga into your life. Downward Dog, Child's Pose, Upward Dog and a "Table Top" on your forearms can help with relieving gas and moving around.

Drink Ginger Tea or Chew on Ginger. Ginger helps stimulate saliva, bile and gastric juice production to aid in digestion. In addition, ginger has muscle relaxant properties that can help relieve gases trapped in a constricted digestive system.

Apple Cider Vinegar. Boost stomach acid to aid in digestion and the breakdown of food around meals. Mix 1 tablespoon of raw, organic, unpasteurized apple cider vinegar with a cup of water or herbal tea.

Sauerkraut, Kefir or Kimchi. Eat 1-2 spoonfuls or 8 oz. of kefir when bloating strikes to help give your body a dose of healthy, gut inflammation-fighting good bacteria.

De-Bloating Supplements
- **Activated Charcoal.** Found in supplement form, activated charcoal is a known gas reliever found over the counter.
- **Atrantil.** A supplement designed with bloating, abdominal discomfort and constipation in mind. Directly relievES the methane-gas production that occurs with bloating. You can order it online at: http://atrantil.com
- **Digestive Enzymes.** Take 1-2 with a meal (either right before or after).
- **Garlic** & **Ginger.** A natural de-bloating effect.
- **Take Bitters & Herbs.** Such as dandelion, chamomile, licorice root and aloe vera. Sold in capsule or tincture form (liquid drops you can put on your tongue to stimulate healthy digestion).
- **Turmeric.** A natural anti-inflammatory sold in powder or condiment form, like a yellow mustard that contains turmeric to keep in the fridge. Take a spoon full at the first sign of bloating (then wash down with a glass of warm water). Or use Liposomal Curcumin.

In-The-Moment-Relief: Constipation (Many of these techniques are similar to de-bloating):

- Sip Dandelion, Peppermint, Ginger and/or Licorice Tea
- Deep breathing 30 seconds (repeat throughout the day—5-10-times)
- Massage your abdomen to stimulate colon
- Get down on all fours, and stick your rump up in the air.
- Take Digestive Enzymes with meals
- Organic Apple Cider Vinegar. Mix one tablespoon with a cup of water or herbal tea.

The 28 Day Gut Kickstart

- Turmeric. Buy a yellow mustard that contains turmeric and take a spoon full.
- Take Your Time to go.
- Castor Oil. Rub on your stomach as a topical substance.
- Chew on ginger or herbs, like dandelion, chamomile, licorice root and aloe vera
- Get a Squatty Potty

Constipation-Relief Supplements

- **Aloe** (soothing effect)
- **Antimicrobial Herbs** (Dysbiocide by Biotics)
- **Beta-TCP (Biotics) or Ox Bile** to support your liver/gallbladder health and function for breaking down fats, creating bile and eliminating wastes and toxins.
- **Bitter Herbs.** Herbal formulas to help stimulate bowels.
- **Peppermint**
- **Magnesium (Ozonated Magnesium, Magnesium Glycinate or Magnesium Citrate)** Try taking it in the evening before bed with extra water for a normal bowel movement in the morning.
- **Micro Emulsified Oregano Tablets**
- **Pre-biotic (Partially Hydrolyzed Guar Gum, Glucomannan) & Probiotic Supplement** (soil-based probiotic)
- **Prokinetic GI Motility Agents.** (Contraindicated with SSRIs)
- **Vitamin-Electrolyte Blends** (Vitamin C, Mg, K, C)
- Other **Essentials to Consider**: Zinc, Vitamin B Complex, Vitamin C, Cod Liver Oil (Also contains: Vitamin D and/or Vitamin A)

Note: ***Don't overdo it.*** *It can be easy to want to do EVERYTHING to relieve bloating and constipation when it strikes. Proceed with caution. If you load up on every remedy under the sun at once, you may end up sending your body out of balance in the other direction.*

GERD

Approximately 1 in 5 people experience GERD or "heart burn" on a regular basis, and a vast majority of these people take a PPI (acid suppressing drug) to help mitigate symptoms.

The problem?

PPI drugs actually make symptoms of GERD worse, not better, in the long term. More and more research now shows that GERD is actually a sign of TOO LITTLE stomach acid (not too much), as well as bacterial overgrowth, and when you have TOO LITTLE stomach acid or TOO MUCH unhealthy bacteria in your gut, your body is unable to digest your food appropriately.

The good news? You can heal from GERD naturally! Here's your cheat sheet protocol:

Step 1: Reduce factors that promote bacterial overgrowth and low stomach acid.

1. **Work with your doctor to titrate off of proton pump inhibitors (PPIs)** and other acid-suppressing drugs (TUMS, Nexium).
2. **Address underlying and correlated gut symptoms including**: chronic stress, H. pylori & other GI infections, pernicious anemia (B12), hypothyroidism, gastritis, and nutrient deficiencies. Work with a functional medicine or nutrition practitioner.
3. **A Low FODMAP Paleo Diet** may also improve symptoms while addressing underlying conditions. Some common HIGH FODMAP foods you may remove include: apples, onions, asparagus, avocado, wheat, dairy, legumes, broccoli, Brussels sprouts, peach, pear, plum, cherry, eggplant, watermelon, cabbage.

Step 2: Replace stomach acid, digestive enzymes, and key nutrients for digestion and health.

1. **Add in "stomach acid."** Take Betaine HCL tablet* (not recommended if still currently on PPIs, pregnant of you have ulcers/gastritis), and/or Take Bitter Herbs, or Apple Cider Vinegar.
2. **Add 1-2 Digestive Enzymes with Meals**. Protease/pepsin, amylase, glucoamylase, lipase, ox bile, etc.
3. **Nutrients**. Assess your need via diet assessment & blood work. These may include niacin, chloride, sodium, potassium, zinc, and iodine
4. Niacin Foods: Chicken, Turkey, Grass-fed Beef, Tuna, Mushrooms, Organ Meats, Green Peas
5. Chloride Foods: Sea Salt, Seaweed/Sea Veggies, Tomatoes, Lettuce, Celery, and Olives.
6. Sodium Foods: Sea Salt
7. Potassium Foods: Bananas, Avocados, Winter Squash, Sweet Potatoes, Coconut Water, Wild Caught Salmon
8. Zinc: Shellfish (oysters, crab, lobsters), Organ Meats, Grass-fed Beef, Chicken, Dark Chocolate
9. Iodine: Sea Vegetables (kelp, kombu, hijiki, arame), Grass-fed Raw Cheese & Dairy, Pastured Eggs, Wild-Caught Fish.

Step 3: Restore beneficial bacteria and a healthy mucosal lining in the gut.

1. Take probiotics, prebiotics, and eat fermented foods, etc.
2. Consider supplements to aid in GI mucosa healing (like **GI Revive** o**r GastroMend** from Designs for Health)

*How much HCL should you take?!
Do the HCL Challenge Test with your tablets to find out how many you need. Before a meal one day, simply take one capsule, wait a minute to see if you experience a warming, burning

sensation. If not, take one more capsule, wait a minute to assess for the same thing. Continue this process until a warming sensation is reached, THEN you know your "optimal" dose for HCL tablets—your ideal dose is the dose you took right BEFORE you reached that warming sensation.

No warmth? Stick to 2-3 capsules with meals. Sometimes when stomach acid is dramatically suppressed or you experience symptoms elsewhere (like a warming sensation in the back of your neck or head), your body can be disconnected with the sensation in your gut. Boost your stomach acid naturally and consistently and natural HCL can be re-won!

IBS/IBD

Irritable Bowel Syndrome (IBS) is often referred to as a syndrome of "exclusion" when no other causes are known as to what drives the symptoms of bloating, constipation and interchanging loose and/or hard-to-pass stools. Nevertheless, it is SUPER uncomfortable and something you DON'T have to live with forever. Whether you experience ongoing constipation or diarrhea, IBS can be reversed with these steps.

Essentials for Treating IBS Naturally
In order to effectively treat IBS, you must:

1. **First test and treat any underlying "pathogens" present** (i.e. parasites, low stomach acid, overgrowth of bad bacteria, SIBO, etc.). The BEST way to identify these pathogens is through testing, including comprehensive stool testing, SIBO breath testing, comprehensive blood work, and potentially food intolerance testing and organic acids (urine testing). Work with a functional medicine or nutrition practitioner familiar in testing and treating these conditions.

2. **Assess other outside "triggers."** Aside from underlying pathogens (such as bacterial overgrowth or parasites) assess what stressors could be driving your condition, like food allergies or intolerances, heavy metal, mold, and toxic exposure, lack of sleep, and chronic stress (HPA axis dysfunction).
3. **Address inflammation.** Once you determine the pathogens and triggers driving your IBS, address these stressors through lifestyle and dietary changes (i.e. managing stress, eliminating foods that make your symptoms worse, detoxing your hygiene and cleaning products, and integrating supplements and herbs to help).

Here are some specific treatments and supplements that can aid in the relief of IBS:

IBS-C (Constipation)
- Get 7-9 hours of sleep (shortened sleep shortens the elimination process)
- Stress Management (doing things you love, sleeping, playing, taking movement breaks, drinking enough water, gut-directed hypnotherapy, yoga, etc.)
- Increase soluble fiber (prebiotics) (i.e. partially hydrolyzed guar gum (PHGG) supplements, and prebiotic foods, like cooked and cooled sweet potatoes/potatoes, carrots, and squashes, green tipped bananas and plantains, and cooked and cooled white rice.

Supplemental Support Options
- **Antimicrobial Herbal Supplements.** Kill off bad gut bacteria.
- **Bitter Herbs:** Take under tongue to stimulate bile (waste) production.
- **GI Renew (Designs for Health).** A blend of herbs to support elimination.

- **Magnesium.** Magnesium Glycinate (200-600 mg/day) [*don't use high doses long term] and Magnesium Citrate plus Calcium relaxes digestive muscles (like Natural Calm, 1-2 tsp. before bed)
- **Ox Bile.** Liver Support to encourage detoxification and proper waste production.
- **Peppermint.** Natural stimulant and soother for constipation.
- **Prebiotics & Probiotics**
- **Prokinetic.** Helps move bowels through.
- **Vitamin-Electrolyte Blends** Vitamin C stimulates digestion.

For bloating symptoms: Atrantil (2 capsules with meals, diminishes bloating as well)

IBS-D (Diarrhea)
- Antimicrobial Herbal Supplements. Kill off bad gut bacteria.
- Atrantil. Diminishes bloating if bloating symptoms are present.
- Bitter Herbs. Calm stomach aggravation or abdominal upset.
- Butyrate Supplement (sodium/potassium form + prebiotic powder in water)
- GAPS or Elemental diet (specifically for Crohn's)
- Ginger & Ginger Tea.
- Peppermint Oil
- Prebiotics
- Probiotics (soil-based)

Best probiotics for diarrhea/loose stools
- Soil-based organisms
- Transient commensals
- Saccharomyces boulardii

- VSL#3
- Elixa

IBD (Irritable Bowel Disease)

IBD includes Crohn's and ulcerative colitis, which are autoimmune diseases wherein the body inappropriately attacks commensal bacteria, leading to altered gut bacteria, inflammation, and intestinal permeability. IBD is thought to be both a byproduct of underlying gut pathogens (like SIBO, low stomach acid, etc.), as well as cause of these things—it is bidirectional.

Protocols look similar to IBS, with a few variations:

Active Flare
- AIP Diet, GAPS Diet, or Low FODMAP Diet
- Antimicrobial Herbs
- Butyrate 3-4 g & Prebiotics
- FMT Fecal Microbiota Transplant
- Probiotics (soil based) & Prebiotics.

Remission/Maintenance
- AIP Diet, GAPS Diet, or Low FODMAP Diet
- Curcumin Supplementation
- Colostrum. Tegricel form best; 1.5 g/day
- Glutathione. Liposomal form best; 2 tsp per day.
- Probiotics & Prebiotics.
- Vitamin D (if low)
- Aim for serum level of 40-60 ng/mL

Leaky Gut

Leaky gut, or intestinal permeability, is a condition or "syndrome" which happens when the tissue lining of your small intestine becomes permeable, weak and "leaky," allowing undigested food particles, bacteria, and toxins into your bloodstream, leading to a potentially outsized immune response.

Leaky gut is NOT a disease or something you're stuck with for life. Instead, it is a byproduct of various stressors (like processed foods and NSAIDs) and "wear and tear" of poor digestion or poor digestive hygiene that occurs over time.

Sort of like what happens if you don't brush your teeth (you get cavities), the same thing goes for your gut health:

If you don't have healthy gut hygiene (like chewing your food well, eating a balance of real whole foods, drinking clean filtered water, probiotics, etc.) and if you don't manage lifestyle stress, then more often than not, you get a leaky gut.

How does this affect you? Inflammation!

If the damage to the lining of your gut is bad enough that such substances regularly leak through, it can wreak havoc on your health.

Common side effects of leaky gut include:

1. Frequent Bloating & Gas
2. Chronic Constipation or "IBS"
3. Loose Stools or Chronic Diarrhea
4. Stomach Pain (particularly after eating)
5. Sugar, Carbohydrate & Coffee Cravings
6. Frequent Headaches and/or Migraines
7. Joints that Pop or Click &/or Arthritis
8. Inability to Hold an Adjustment or Heal Muscle Tissue
9. Craving Foods that don't make you feel well
10. Allergies (food and/or seasonal and environmental)
11. Acne https://drlauryn.com/adult-acne/ , Skin Breakouts & Rashes (Eczema, whiteheads, etc.)
12. Autoimmune Conditions and Cancer

13. High Cholesterol Markers (even with "healthy eating")
14. Easily Sick or Run Down
15. Low Energy (despite sleeping) https://drlauryn.com/adrenal-fatigue/
16. Anxiety https://drlauryn.com/cure-anxiety-naturally/ , Depression, ADD/ADHD
17. Autism Spectrum Disorder & Neurological Disorders
18. Dental Cavities
19. Diabetes or Blood Sugar Imbalances (hypo/hyperglycemia)
20. Hormone Imbalances (infertility, amenorrhea, horrible PMS or menopause, PCOS)

WHAT TO DO ABOUT IT?!

First and foremost, building a base of a "healthy gut" maintenance plan and diminished lifestyle stress is key including:

- Awareness of your underlying gut pathogens or conditions driving your leaky gut (SIBO, low stomach acid, fungal overgrowth or infection, HPA Axis Dysfunction)
- Nutrient-dense whole-foods diet
- Daily stress busting practices
- Probiotics AND prebiotics

Once you have this foundation laid, you can start integrating and experimenting with these magic ingredients:

- **Apple Cider Vinegar.** A natural stomach acid booster that promotes healthy stomach acid to help fully digest foods (and prevent undigested food particles from leaking into your bloodstream). Consume one tbsp. in 2-4 oz. of water with meals.
- **Butyrate Supplementation**. In addition to fermentable fiber, which contains butyrate, butyrate supplementation appears to play an especially important role in regulating

barrier function (Peng et al, 2009 https://www.ncbi.nlm.nih.gov/pmc/articles/PMC2728689/). Low butyrate causes tight intestinal junction lesions (holes) and impaired intestinal permeability. Try: One dose Sodium-Potassium Butyrate (not Cal-Mag) http://amzn.to/2HLbku6.
- **Colostrum**. A natural component of breast milk best known for its probiotic and powerful gut healing effects. As an adult, its available in supplemental form and has been shown to decrease intestinal permeability—even in athletes who maintain physically stressful lifestyles (Halasa et al, 2017 https://www.ncbi.nlm.nih.gov/pubmed/28397754). Try: ProSerum whey by Well Wisdom http://amzn.to/2IB3BAb . 1 Serving Daily.
- **Glutamine**. An amino acid known for repairing the gut lining. Consume 20-40 mg. per day in water. Try: Enteromend by Thorne http://amzn.to/2G89pTm . 1-3 servings daily.
- **Probiotics & Prebiotics.** These two are staples in any gut-loving plan.
- **Vitamins A & D.** Vitamin A manages the growth and differentiation of intestinal cells. Deficiencies in Vitamin A has been shown to cause alterations in commensal bacteria and to impair the gut barrier (Lima et al, 2010 https://www.ncbi.nlm.nih.gov/pmc/articles/PMC2830290/). Additionally, Vitamin D, another fat-soluble vitamin, also plays a role in gut barrier function. Vitamin D deficiency is correlated with inflammatory bowel disease and intestinal permeability (Assa et al, 2014 https://academic.oup.com/jid/article/210/8/1296/2911874) (Ananthakrishnan, 2016 https://www.ncbi.nlm.nih.gov/pmc/articles/PMC5114499/) . Try: Cod liver oil—more absorbable than the synthetic formulas of Vitamin A and Vitamin

D supplements. I like Rosita Cod Liver Oil https://www.corganic.com/products/evclo#592254c4b8e65 capsules.
- **Zinc.** Helps maintain intestinal integrity as it is a vital component in practically every cell in our body (Skrovanek et al, 2014 https://www.ncbi.nlm.nih.gov/pmc/articles/PMC4231515/). Take up to 110 mg/day for a short-term therapeutic trial (no more than 8 weeks) Try Biotics Aqueous Zinc http://amzn.to/2HN8lBF for 7 days, then switch to a capsule form like this one https://www.purecapspro.com/drlauryn/pe/products/product_details.asp?ProductsID=1003

Liver/Gallbladder Dysfunction

Your liver is the organ responsible for detoxification in your body. If it is under functioning, then your body is at risk for toxic burden in your body, as well as impaired gallbladder function (the organ responsible for creating bile to help break down fats in the small intestine). Symptoms of a "dysfunctional liver" or gallbladder are vast—they include:

External signs:

- Coated tongue
- Bad breath
- Red palms and soles
- Flushed facial appearance or excessive facial blood vessels (capillaries/veins)
- Acne, Rosacea
- Yellow conjunctiva on the eyes
- Red swollen itchy eyes (allergic eyes)
- Dark circles under the eyes
- Brownish spots and blemishes on the skin (liver spots)
- Rashes and itchy skin (pruritus)

Abnormal breakdown of fats (lipids) leading to:

- Abnormalities in the level of fats in the blood stream e.g. elevated LDL cholesterol and reduced HDL cholesterol and elevated triglycerides.
- Arteries blocked with fat, leading to high blood pressure, heart attacks and strokes.
- Fatty liver and build up of fat in other body organs.
- Obesity and/or inability to lose weight
- Sluggish metabolism

Along with other similar sounding symptoms:

- Allergies: sinus, hay fever, asthma, dermatitis, hives, etc.
- Skin rashes and inflammations
- Chemical and food sensitivities
- Autoimmune diseases
- Chronic Fatigue Syndrome and Fibromyalgia
- Recurrent viral, bacterial and parasitic infections
- Blood sugar problems
- Hormonal imbalances
- Mood swings
- Poor concentration/brain fog
- Depression
- Headaches

Phew! That's A LOT of symptoms.

How to heal and strengthen your liver or gallbladder?

Juice fasts and "liver cleanses" are popular in the mainstream, but loving your liver goes far beyond sipping green juice.

Here are supportive measures you can take to make your most primary detoxification organ and its second-mate (gallbladder) work well:

- Refrain from NSAID use and any other unnecessary medications
- Quit smoking or drinking alcohol in excess
- Sip dandelion tea
- Try a coffee enema if you experience nausea or other gut symptoms that don't seem like they improve with gut support alone. (Use caution: Some people become addicted to the use of coffee enemas—almost relying on them to be able to go. Continue to support your gut health and dig deeper below the surface, potentially treating for gut dysbiosis or bacterial overgrowth if warranted)
- Incorporate raw vegetable juice in morning
- Apple Cider
- Consider getting a metal/liver toxicity screening
- **Eat**: Beets, artichokes, chia seeds and flax seeds, grapefruits, apples, spinach and leafy greens (dark), liver and organ meats, blueberries, cold-water fatty fish, lemons, onions, garlic, Cruciferous vegetables such as cauliflower, broccoli, cabbage, Brussels sprouts, Bok Choy, kale, radishes, and turnips (contain glucosinolates which help the liver produce enzymes for detoxification); Bitter vegetables such as bitter gourd, dandelion greens, mustard greens and chicory (promote the production and flow of bile).

Supplemental Support
- Herbs which cleanse the liver (Turmeric, Amalaki, Guduchi, Barberry, Bhumyamalaki, Milk Thistle, Dandelion)
- Beet juice
- Taurine (Beta TCP)
- Vitamins C and E and beta carotene.

- Adrenal health support (HPA Balance)
- Vitamin B Complex
- Cod Liver Oil

Nutrient Deficiencies

Malabsorption (i.e. leaky gut) of nutrients can lead to nutrient deficiencies simply because you are not getting what you need. From iron deficiencies, to Vitamin B, C, D, Magnesium, and Zinc. While the nutrients are unique to you and vast, the bottom line is something is *leaky* in your raft, and no matter how many supplements you take with these missing nutrients, you will not absorb them, unless you first heal and repair your gut.

- **Eat** real whole, **colorful** (nutrient dense) foods—aim for 3-5 different colors at least, including in-season produce and sustainably raised meats
- **Apple Cider Vinegar** to enhance stomach acid if needed
- **Drink warm liquids** before meals
- **Avoid drinking cold water** during meals (stalls digestion)
- **Avoid iron/copper in supplements** and multivitamins (unless severe iron deficiency is present)

Aim to get missing nutrients first through foods, and single doses of supplements—as opposed to a multi-vitamin, such as:

Antioxidants. Fight "free radicals" or stress. Boost energy. Eat in-season, colorful fruits and veggies including wild blueberries, Goji Berries, spinach, dark chocolate, raw pecans, artichokes, cranberries, elderberries, tomatoes, carrots, pumpkin seeds, sweet potatoes, pomegranates, strawberries, kale, broccoli, grapes, squash, wild-caught salmon.and herbs (bilberry, turmeric, grape seed, pine bark, ginkgo biloba).

B-Vitamins. Metabolic functions, carbohydrate utilization, hydrochloric acid production, enzyme function and energy.   Eat sustainably raised meats and cold water fatty fish, nutritional yeast, and grass-fed cheese.

Calcium: Bone health and muscle contractions. Eat: Spinach & Leafy Greens, Broccoli, Brussels Sprouts, Raw Almonds, Organic Goat's Milk. Don't take calcium supplements, but instead Magnesium, Vitamin A & D to boost absorption.

Iodine: Thyroid support and function. Eat: Iodized salts, kelp granules, organ meats, cold-water carry fish.

Iron: Makes and oxygenates red blood cells. Gives you energy. Eat: Organ meats, sustainably raised meats, spinach and dark leafy greens.

Magnesium: Ease constipation and bloating. Healthy muscle relaxation. Eat: Dark chocolate, dark leafy greens, raw nuts and seeds.

Vitamin A: Boosts your immune system, skin health and vision, plus aids in absorption of healthy fats. Eat: Organ meats, extra virgin cod liver oil, sweet potatoes, carrots.

Vitamin C: Boosts your immune system. Eat: Citrus, berries, leafy greens, broccoli, Brussels Sprouts.

Vitamin D: Aid in absorption calcium, positive mood, bone growth, absorption of healthy fats and energy. Eat: Cold water fatty fish, pastured egg yolks, sardines, organic organ meats, full-fat grass-fed dairy (if tolerated), extra-virgin cod-liver oil. Aim for 30-60 minutes sun exposure daily.

Supplement Support:
- Licorice Root
- L-Glutamine
- Pre-biotics or Jerusalem Artichoke (Helianthus tuberosus) (tuber) *
- Digestive Enzymes

- Cod Liver Oil
- Fiber
- Zinc + Zinc-Carnosine (promotes a healthy gastric microbial balance and helps maintain the integrity of the protective gastric mucosal lining by supporting healthy mucus secretion)

SIBO

SIBO, or "Small intestinal bacterial overgrowth", is the overgrowth of bacteria from the large intestine into the small intestine.

While it's important to note that **ALL healthy guts have bacteria—both "good" and "bad,"** Good bacteria helps your gut do things like: Protect against other "bad" bacteria and yeast, absorb nutrients and vitamins, and maintain the motility of digestion. Too much bacteria in your large intestine (and eventually your small intestine) leads to perpetual issues like:

- Bloating, constipation, and gas
- IBS
- Autoimmune conditions
- Adrenal distress
- Allergies
- Mood swings
- Anxiety and depression (brain gut connection)
- Hormonal Imbalances
- ADD/ADHD
- Thyroid imbalances
- Infertility
- Difficult focusing
- Low energy
- Blood sugar highs and lows

Enter: SIBO.

SIBO is bacterial overgrowth in the small intestine which doesn't just go away overnight—it consists of bacteria lingering in your gut that triggers a host of imbalances in the body (both in the gut and connected to the gut).

HOW TO GET RID OF IT

SIBO is a stubborn pathology that requires a targeted gut support protocol to eradicate it, namely through botanical/antimicrobial treatment, diet and lifestyle support. SIBO is notorious for coming back with vengeance, so give your protocol at least 30-60 days.

The cool thing about SIBO is if you suspect you have it, you can treat it as if you do. If symptoms improve, then treatment was warranted and effective.

On top of your basic digestive protocol and real-foods diet, here are some suggestions for "beating" SIBO:

1. Eat a Balance of Proteins, Fats & Carbs.
Yes, continue to eat carbohydrates while on your SIBO protocol. Contrary to popular belief, a low FODMAP diet (low carb diet) is not necessarily necessary, and moderate amounts of carbohydrates, in conjunction with your SIBO supplements can actually help eliminate the overgrowth of bacteria faster. In addition, SIBO can also feed off ketones (fatty acids produced on a low-carb diet). Eat foods that make you feel good.

2. **Incorporate** soil-based organism probiotics and transit commensal organisms (see suggestions below).

3. **Follow the following SIBO supplement protocol for 60-90 days**, then re-test if you had testing done

SIBO Supplement Protocol

It may seem like alot, but that bacteria will not know what hit 'em!

Morning:
- Soil-based Organism Probiotic
- Anti-Biofilm Enzyme Klaire Labs: Interfase Plus

Breakfast:
- Ox Bile
- HCL or Apple Cider Vinegar
- Monolaurin Lauricidin- 1 scoop
- Antimicrobials Biotics: Dysbiocide + FC Cidal, or Metagenics: Candida-AR + Candida BR
- Digestive Enzymes x 1 Transformation Enzymes: Digest or Designs for Health: Digestzymes
- HCL x 1-2 Metagenics: Metagest or Biotics: Betaine Plus HP

Noon:
- Transit Commensal Organism Probiotic Megaspore
- Monolaurin Lauricidin
- Digestive Enzymes x 1
- HCL x 1-2

Afternoon:
- Anti-Biofilm Enzyme Klaire Labs: Interfase Plus

Night:
- Monolaurin Lauricidin- 1 scoop
- Antimicrobials Biotics: Dysbiocide + FC Cidal, or Metagenics: Candida-AR + Candida BR
- Digestive Enzymes x 1 Transformation Enzymes: Digest or Designs for Health: Digestzymes
- HCL x 1-2 Metagenics: Metagest or Biotics: Betaine Plus HP

Before Bed:
Soil-Based Probiotic Megaspore

Additional Support

- Atrantil (If you do not partake in the full SIBO protocol, this supplement is a good "first step" for banishing bloating; good for methane-provoked SIBO)
- Cod Liver Oil
- Digestive Bitters (help with constipation)
- Peppermint Oil
- Prokinetic (improves motility of GI; Pure Encapsulations: MotilPro)
- Zinc (Heal & Seal Gut)

Skin Conditions

50 percent of **adult** women and 25 percent of **adult** men have acne at some point in their adult lives. Acne and skin conditions are directly related to your gut health, and are generally an autoimmune or inflammatory reaction, letting you know something is going on inside.

In addition, your skin eats what you eat *and* also what you put on it. If you're using products with foreign chemicals and unwanted toxins, your body (and gut) can get stressed out—and pimples will let you know all about it.

Never fear!

Clear your skin with a few of these slight edges (Bonus: If you have allergies, these remedies will help those, too):

Beauty Foods

1. Beets
2. Berries

3. Butternut Squash
4. Chia Seeds
5. Coconut Kefir
6. Coconut Oil
7. Collagen & Gelatin
8. Extra Virgin Olive Oil
9. Fermented Foods
10. Kefir (Goats Milk, Coconut, Water)
11. Leafy Greens
12. Pastured Egg Yolks
13. Pastured, Organic & Sustainably Raised Meats (not conventional)
14. Pomegranate
15. Pumpkin
16. Organ Meats
17. Raw Almonds
18. Spirulina
19. Walnuts
20. Wild-Caught Fatty Fish (Salmon, Tuna, Mackerel, Sardines)

Avoid: *Dairy, grains, corn, soy, sugar, legumes, hydrogenated vegetable oils*

Nutrient & Vitamin Boosters

Take Apple Cider Vinegar or HCL. 1 tbsp. in 2-4 oz. of water 2-3 times each day to boost natural acidity of your GI system.

Biotin. Fresh renewed skin is yours.

Collagen Protein & Bone Broth. Heal and seal the gut.

Herbal Antihistamines. Fights against histamine response in your gut that triggers poor skin health.

Niacin. Prevents skin dryness and rashes.

Vitamin A. Promotes new cells and healthy immunity. Deficiency Signs: Rough, dry Skin
Find in: Cod Liver Oil (1-2 tsp/day), Liver, Kidney, Other Organ Meats, Grass-Fed Dairy, Carrots, Bell Peppers, Sweet Potatoes, Dark Leafy Greens, Winter Squash, Cantaloupe

Vitamin C. Essential for healthy collagen in skin (helps protect against wrinkles and keratinization-hardening of skin)
Find In: Spinach & other Dark Leafy Greens, Citrus fruits, Bell Peppers, Broccoli, Brussels Sprouts, Kiwi, Strawberries, supplements

Vitamin E & K2. Fat soluble vitamins that increases hydration and natural anti-inflammation.

Silica. Skin hydration and tautness.

Zinc. Promotes good skin immunity and wound healing, as well as protects against UV radiation and inflammation. Heals and seals the gut lining.

Find In: Spinach, Shellfish (Shrimp, Oysters), Grass-Fed Bison & Beef, Flax Seeds, Kidney Beans, Pastured Egg Yolks, Wild-Caught Salmon, Pastured Turkey, Organic Chicken, Cocoa powder, Supplement (10-15 mg/day)

Beautify

Change up the skin care and hygiene products you buy. Throw out any conventional products with parabens, sulfates and other toxic chemicals. Putting chemicals on your body will limit your skin's natural healing processes. Instead try: Majestically Made, Beautycounter, Skin Foodie, FatCo, The Dirt, Primal Life Organics.

Make your own homemade skin care!

- **Coconut Oil.** Use **coconut oil on both your skin and in your hair** to help cleanse, moisturize, remove makeup, heal wounds or scars quicker, and prevent razor burn.
- **Tea Tree Oil.** Fight breakouts, redness and inflammation on the skin.
- **Jojoba Oil.** Natural moisturizer.
- **Avocado & Avocado Oil.** Vitamins A, D and E penetrate the skin.
- **Sea Salt.** Protects, tightens and restores skin.
- **Apple Cider Vinegar.** Kills pathogens (like bacteria) and clears up skin problems caused by gut issues,
- **Raw Honey.** Reduces breakouts, moistures moisturizing properties, assists wound healing, fights off allergies or rashes, and antiseptic properties help reduce scars.
- Other Moisturizing Agents
    - ▷ Shea Butter
    - ▷ Aloe
    - ▷ Almond Oil
    - ▷ Argan Oil
    - ▷ Lemon Oil

Detox 101

"Never go to a doctor whose office plants have died."

In other words: Health goes beyond what we feed our bodies, but is also in how we *treat* our bodies and *interact* with our environments.

Get this: Your body eats what your skin eats.

When you feed your skin toxic chemicals and interact with chemicals and toxins in your daily environment, your body does not eat good things.

Beauty Product 101

Beauty products, toiletries, household cleaners and even our own water sources are a major source of chemical exposure for a lot of people.

Here are a few chemicals in many hair products, soaps and cosmetics that line the shelves of Target, Wal-Mart, and yes, Sephora, includes:

- **BHA and BHT :** Used mainly in moisturizers and make-up as preservatives. Suspected cancer-causing agents and endocrine disruptors. In fact, high doses of BHT may mimic estrogen, the primary female sex hormone, and prevent expression of male sex hormones (testosterone), resulting in adverse reproductive effects. Long-term exposure to high doses of BHT has also proven toxic in mice and rats, causing liver, thyroid and kidney problems and affecting lung function and blood coagulation.
- **Sodium Lauryl Sulfate**: A toxic detergent found in most shampoos, soaps and toothpastes. It absorbs very readily through mucous membranes and is linked to skin irritation (dandruff, canker sores, dermatitis), as well as a known penetration enhancer—helping other harsh chemicals get into your body. It is actually also commonly used to kill plants and insects.
- **Lead**: Known carcinogen found in lipstick and hair dye, but never listed because it's a contaminant, not an ingredient.
- **Mercury**: Known allergen which impairs brain development. Found in mascara and some eye drops.
- **Talc**: Similar to asbestos in composition, it's found in baby powder, eye shadow, blush, and deodorant. Linked to ovarian cancer and respiratory problems.

No, you don't have to live in a bubble…**But if you wouldn't feed your bod a steady diet of fast food, sugar, fake and processed foods—why would you do the same to your body, face, and hair?**

And why would you want to touch something, wear something, or spray something near you that is poisonous to your body?

Stop polluting your body!

How to Detox

We often associate the word "detox" with green juice cleanses, bone broth and laxatives. But "detoxing" goes beyond juicing, coffee enemas and liquid-only diets.

It also spans the products we use on our skin, in our house and in our daily beauty routine.

In light of a new, healthy, more thriving you, consider giving your beauty kit, toiletry items and household cleaners an overhaul.

The trick to protecting your health and not breaking the bank?

Start with a few things—perhaps the things you use most, like a natural, chemical-free countertop spray and dishwasher detergent, some new foundation (Josie Maran's foundation with argan oil is amazing!) and a face wash that energizes your skin (and doesn't clog it with toxic chemicals).

Take Action

Look into starting small—and replacing one beauty product, makeup or hygiene product you've been using with a homemade or organic, non-toxic version.

Here are some homemade recipes for beauty and homecare, as well as some makeup, skin-care and cleaner recommendations, and in addition, the **Environmental Working Group's website** is a hub for TONS of information on "best" products, foods and more to pick and choose for your best health (www.ewg.com) and the **Think Dirty app** will give you the dirt on almost any makeup and cleaning product you're thinking of buying.

HOMEMADE BEAUTY RECIPES

Homemade Toothpaste

Ingredients
- 2/3 cup baking soda
- 1 tsp fine sea salt
- 1 – 2 tsp peppermint extract or 10-15 drops peppermint oil
- filtered water

Directions
When you are ready to brush, simply wet your toothbrush, scoop or spread as much paste as you like and begin brushing.

Natural Makeup Remover

Plain olive or coconut oil are great for removing mascara (even waterproof) and will remove other makeup as well, but isn't as ideal if you have oily skin.

For oily skin: Use pure, organic Liquid Castille in water will remove makeup without adding oils to the skin or stripping the natural ones. A few drops on a washcloth or in a sink full of water will naturally clean your face.

Banana-Apple Cider Mask (*acne/blemish fighter)

Ingredients
1/2 small banana, mashed
2 tablespoons Apple Cider Vinegar
1 teaspoon raw honey
2 tablespoons yogurt

Directions:
Simply combine all the ingredients in a bowl. Apply a thin layer to your face then relax for up to 20 minutes. Rinse the mask off with warm water, then apply your favorite moisturizer.

Gentle Face Cleansing

Ingredients
- 3 Tbsp Organic Extra virgin Coconut oil
- 1 tsp Raw Honey
- 1 tsp Baking Soda (gently exfoliates, draws out toxins)

Directions
- Put coconut oil and honey in a small bowl and stir well with a spoon.
- Add baking soda and stir in very well.
- Spoon into a clean container with lid.
- Store at room temperature.
- No worries if if hardens, it will melt when applied to skin from your body heat.

Ghee Skincare Moisturizer

Ingredients
- 1/4 cup ghee
- 2.5 tsp olive oil
- 2-3 drops of essential oil (like lavender)

Directions
- Melt the fat in the microwave in a glass container.
- Stir in the olive oil and essential oil.
- Refrigerate, uncovered, until the balm hardens.
- Remove from the refrigerator and store tightly.
- Use on face post-cleansing or all over body like lotion

Facial Toner

Ingredients
- Filtered water
- Raw apple cider vinegar
- Lavender essential oil
- Or, Frankincense essential oil

Directions
- For normal to dry skin, mix 1/3 part vinegar to 2/3 part filtered water. Add a few drops of Lavender or Frankincense oils.
- For oily and acne-prone skin, mix 1/2 part vinegar and 1/2 part filtered water. Add a few drops of lavender or frankincense oils.
- Store in a container or bottle at room temperature.
- Use twice a day – first thing in the morning and right before bed.

SKIN & MAKEUP RECOMMENDATIONS

Makeup:
Araza Beauty
Beautycounter
Primal Life Organics
Josie Maran
100% Pure

Skin & Body:
Ecology Skincare
Fat Face Skin Co. (Skin care & Deodorant)
The Dirt (toothpaste, deodorant)
Pacifica
Skin Foodie (All body care)
JASON Brand (Shampoo, Conditioner, Body Wash)
Seabreeze (Shampoo, Conditioner, Body Wash)

HOMEMADE HOUSEHOLD CLEANERS

Sometimes the purest, simplest, most effective and most cost effective cleaners are items you probably already have already the house:

- **Lemon juice and vinegar:** Lemons are great for cleaning windows and cutting through grease, and vinegar is useful for preventing mold.
- **Table salt** (or sea salt) is great for scrubbing and scouring tough dirt and grime and for helping to disinfect high traffic areas.
- **Baking Soda:** Natural household cleaning! It scrubs and scours, cleanses, deodorizes, and even helps unclog drains when mixed with vinegar.

Here are 8 awesome recipes for DIY home cleaning agents you can make yourself on the cheap:
Shopping List:
Baking Soda
Distilled White Vinegar
Hydrogen Peroxide
Castile Soap (like Dr. Bronner's)
Essential Oil(s) of choice: Tea Tree, Peppermint, Orange

Natural Salt
Lemons
Borax

KITCHEN

1. All Purpose Cleaner

Ingredients
1 cup white vinegar
2 cups water
1 tablespoon castile soap
3-4 drops essential oil

Directions
Combine all of the ingredients in a spray bottle.

2. Tile & Grout Cleaner

Ingredients
1/4 cup water
6 Tablespoons Baking Soda

Directions
Mix water with baking soda into a paste. Apply to grout and let sit, scrub with toothbrush, remove with sponge. (May also lay out baking soda, then spritz with Hydrogen Peroxide and scrub).

3. Floor Cleaner

Ingredients
White Vinegar

Oranges or Lemon

Directions
Fill a jar with (organic) citrus peels and pour undiluted white vinegar over them. Leave for a few days (up to two weeks) and strain out the vinegar to use as a natural cleaner. Break out the Swiffer or rag and scrub, scrub, scrub.
Other Option: Mix 1 cup vinegar in a gallon of water.

4. Oven Cleaning

Ingredients
Baking Soda
Water

Directions
Spray water over the bottom of the oven and dump lots of baking soda (1/4-1/2 inch think) and then spray with more water to make a paste. Leave overnight, then the next day, scrape out all the baking soda mixture and use a wire brush or dish scrubber to scrub any tough spots. After all the baking soda has been wiped off, a vinegar and water rinse will leave a spot free shine.

BATHROOM

5. Toilet Bowl Cleaner

Ingredients
1-2 cups white vinegar

Directions
Use undiluted white vinegar, pour around the top of the toilet bowl, scrub until clean.

6. Sink & Shower Cleaner

Ingredients
1 cup baking soda
½ cup castile soap
3-4 drops essential oil

Directions
Place the baking soda in a bowl. Slowly add the soap until the mixture gets thick. Add in a few drops of an antibacterial essential oil.

7. Drain-O

Ingredients
½ baking soda
½ cup white vinegar
Hot water

Directions
Pour the baking soda down the clogged drain. Follow with vinegar. Allow to fizz for about 10 minutes. Then pour a kettle full of boiling hot water down the drain. Repeat with more water if necessary.

8. Natural Windex

Ingredients
White vinegar
Newspaper

Directions
Spritz white vinegar on mirror and wipe with newspaper.

STORE BOUGHT HOUSEHOLD CLEANERS

It can be overwhelming to decide what products to buy if you hit the store. Here are a few things to keep in mind:

- Be wary of superficially labeled products; start making it a habit to take a closer look at cleaners labeled with the terms "natural," "safe," non-toxic," and "green."
- Buy from reputable companies
- Avoid any products with warnings such as "fatal if inhaled," "poison," "fatal," and vague terms like "surfactant" or "solvent."

Here are some brands to check out:

All Purpose

- Whole Foods 365 Brand (Countertop Cleaners, Laundry Detergent & Dish Soap)
- Dr. Bronner's Organic Pure Castille Soap (all purpose cleaning)
- Dr. Bronner Sal Suds Concentrate (1 tsp + quart of water=surface cleaner and stain treatment)
- Bon Ami Powder (get grime off surfaces)
- Seventh Generation

Dish Soap

- Seventh Generation (Dish detergent, Dish Soap)
- EcoMe Dish Soap
- Ecover Zero Dish Soap
- Biokleen Dish Soap

Laundry

- Seventh Generation (Laundry detergent, Dish Soap)
- Ecover Zero
- Bioklean Laundry Detergent

FAQS

My body feels at war with itself—even though I eat healthy! I don't get why I am still constipated or bloated! What gives?!
The struggle is real! "Healthy eating" can hurt—no matter how clean you keep it. If you find yourself struggling (even when you eat "clean" or try the Refresh Phase part of your program, it is indicative that something is going on "under the hood." And although many foods are healthy, some may not be healthy for you right now. Foods like raw vegetables, green juices, bone broths, eggs and more can be inflammatory for some (no matter how healthy they are) if you have bacterial overgrowth, intestinal permeability, parasites, or more.

Use this book for guidance in digging into what that is through lab testing and working with a practitioner who understands gut healing. Additionally, don't discount the lifestyle factors that also compliment a "healthy" diet—including sleep, stress management, movement, positive mindset and *self-love*.

How does reintroduction work during the Experiment Phase?
One thing at a time. As you reintroduce and try foods during Weeks 5 & 6 with your mindfulness cap on, it is recommended you try one to two new foods at a time in three day increments instead of all at once. This way, you're able to get a clearer perspective around how your gut and body respond (for instance: coffee in the morning three days in a row, followed by steel-cut gluten free oats or eggs and some red pepper flakes with your dinner on day 4-6, then adding back some dark chocolate and hummus with a snack during days 7-9, and so on. You don't have

to experiment with every single food—but you have liberty to be your own experiment.

What if I mess up?
No such thing. Unlike many other programs, "mess ups" don't exist (and no one can force you to do anything). You, my friend, have the power of choice, and, accordingly, you have the freedom to not be perfect. That said, any recommendations given are meant to provide the best opportunity for a clearer picture in your own gut healing journey.

Should I eat 3 or 6 meals day?
It's a longstanding debate without a clear answer: 3 vs. 6 meals per day…which is better?
Ask a personal trainer at Gold's Gym and chances are, he'll tell you: "Eat six small meals per day." Look to *Women's Health* magazine or Dr. Google for a revving metabolism, and chances are, you'll hear the same thing. But then again, three square meals per day is also the human standard—at least culturally speaking: Breakfast, Lunch and Dinner works for many people too.

Should you or shouldn't you snack? Answer: It all depends. Snacking is **NOT** a bad thing, however, when it turns into one of these 3 issues: emotional eating, habitual eating or blood sugar imbalances, it's important to check-in with ourselves:

Am I snacking emotionally or habitually?
And, *Am I eating enough?*

When and if we **eat enough** for our body throughout the day, our body gets the fuel it needs and has less demand on our blood sugar levels to need snacks to make it through the day.

We stay fuller for longer and train our energy systems to run off of fats (granted we are eating fat) over sugar—giving us longer-lasting energy overall. We also allow our digestive system

enough time to process our last meal with less frequent habitual snacking, allowing for all around better digestion and absorption of our nutrients as the digestive system can fully push food through the small intestine in order to make room for the next food into the pipeline.

Again, snacking is NOT a bad thing (and there WILL be times and days when snacking is necessary), but if we are consistently finding ourselves hungry, hangry, or with headaches or low energy levels between meals, we may need to check in with ourselves on if we are truly fueling our body appropriately—whether that means three meals per day plus one snack, six mini meals or three balanced meals, be your own experiment. From a digestive perspective, giving your body time between meals to digest (as long as you're eating enough energy) is golden.

Why no nuts or beans during the 28 day Gut Kickstart? I thought they were healthy…
The Refresh Phase is a 28-day reset for your body and your gut to decide what foods do and do not agree with you. It encourages you eat (in abundance) foods which are commonly easier to digest for the majority of people. All *real* foods (nuts, beans and *some* grains included) can be a totally healthy part of your diet! (and during your Experiment Phase you will get to reintroduce them).

Since nuts and legumes contain Phytic-acid and lectins ("anti-nutrients") on their outer shell, though, they can be more difficult to digest if your gut is already "leaky" or if you've been struggling with digestion. These components help protect plants (like nuts) in the wild from being eaten by predators, wind, storms and other threats and your body sees them like "steel bullets" in your gut (hard to break down) leading to "nut gut" or "bean bloat" in some (i.e. constipation, bloating, brain fog, etc.). In fact, Phytic-acid and lectin are called "anti-nutrients" as well, because they actually bind to vitamins and minerals and make them non-absorbable in your gut. Take a break for 21 days, then by all means, experiment. See how you feel.

Is red meat good or bad?
Sustainability raised red meat is great for you! It is packed with nutrients like iron, protein and Omega-3 fatty acids. Since proteins like red meat and pork take longer to break down, though (approximately 3-5 hours), for 21 days while you reset your gut, it's recommended for you to reach for quicker digesting proteins like chicken, fish and turkey. Contrary to popular belief, grass-fed red meat does not cause high cholesterol, heart disease or cancer, but actually boosts body composition, builds lean muscle, and supplies your body with a nutrient-dense vitamins and minerals. (The same thing goes for butter, full-fat dairy and egg yolks. The real deal healthy fats in these foods actually lessen inflammation—instead of increasing it. Sugar, refined foods and low fat diets are actually the bigger culprits in heart disease, high cholesterol and cancer).

Can I eat egg whites?
Egg whites *and* eggs are not recommended during your 21-day Refresh Phase since most people who do have egg sensitivities are actually intolerant to the egg whites—not the yolks. For others with gut sensitivities or imbalances as well, eggs themselves can trigger bloating, constipation or other gut-related symptoms. For this reason, eggs join the list of the handful of allergenic or gut-irritating foods to take a short break from then to experiment with (in abundance) during your Experiment Phase.

What's the low down on whole grains?
Like nuts and beans, grains—even whole grains—contain Phytic-acid and lectin on their outer shell, along with other components like gluten and gluten-cross contaminating proteins that

also wreak havoc on our gut lining. There is no nutrient found in grains that you can't get from other (real) foods—like veggies, starchy veggies and fruits. During the Experiment Phase, it's encouraged (once again) that you see for yourself and opt for soaked and sprouted grains if you do experiment.

People say gluten is "gut irritating," but why?
Gluten is a protein found in grains like wheat, barley, and rye. It acts as a "glue" in foods with these wheat ingredients (such as cereal, bread, and pasta), helping them hold their shape. When we eat gluten, our body has difficulty digesting the glue-like substance. Gluten is most known for its connection to Celiac disease—an autoimmune disease characterized by an intolerance to gluten. If an individual with Celiac eats gluten, then they are at risk for bloating, IBS, and constipation, as well as a damaged gut lining and intestine. Gluten is a highly inflammatory substance for those without Celiac as well (especially if you have other "gut issues" going on)—particularly in the current processed form that most grains are consumed nowadays (even whole grains). Common signs of gluten intolerance include gas, bloating, constipation, leaky gut, inflammation, autoimmune conditions, arthritis, brain fog, ADD/ADHD, skin breakouts, allergies (seasonal and food), low immunity, hormone imbalances, and chronic conditions (like heart disease, diabetes, Alzheimer's etc.). In fact, with so many signs and symptoms, 1 in 2 people with Celiac themselves do not know they have Celiac.

What about gluten-free grains and products?
The one ingredient missing? Gluten. In the majority of processed food items on the shelves, the foods are just as processed, and many of them contain gluten cross-reactive proteins that trigger similar (gut-irritating) reactions, including: Corn, soy, coffee, quinoa, tapioca, rice, dairy, oats, millet, whey, egg, rye, barley,

spelt, sorghum, yeast, hemp, sesame, amaranth, and potato starch.

You're telling me coffee is a gluten-like substance?
Yes, coffee is one of the highest cross-contaminating foods with gluten—namely instant coffee and poorer quality coffee (like Starbucks and Folgers in your cup). Coffee is also one of the moldiest, most toxic foods we can consume. There are more chemicals in coffee than on an average pharmacy shelf. The majority of coffee beans are contaminated with mycotoxins—damaging compounds created by molds which grow on coffee beans, connected to brain damage, kidney disease, heart conditions and bitter coffee. For this reason, during your 21-day Refresh, it's advised you give yourself a break. Not to mention the fact that this may also provide you with the opportunity to learn to poop on your own (many folks rely on coffee in order to go in the mornings). As you reintroduce coffee, be picky: Choose a fresh, organic quality roast and enjoy one cup if you wish with your add-ins of choice (grass-fed butter, MCT oil, goat's milk kefir, unsweetened almond milk, coconut milk, etc.)

Some people say "low-fat dairy" helps build strong bones and lose weight, others say "dairy makes you break out and get constipated"…Who's right?
Dairy—full-fat grass-fed dairy (the real deal) does do some body's good. In fact, when you reach for the real deal source (full-fat, grass-fed), you actually get less lactose, sugar and more nutrients than low-fat or fat-free processed versions including:

Healthy fats (Saturated and Omega-3's imperative for proper digestion, heart health, cell health, clear skin, nail and hair health, taste, metabolic balance

Vitamin D (absorption of vitamins, minerals and nutrients in the first place)

Vitamin A (vision, immune health, normal growth and development of body tissue)

Calcium that is ACTUALLY absorbed (you need fat-soluble vitamins, like Vitamin D, found in healthy fat, to absorb it)

Probiotics (the **FULL-FAT**, organic, plain versions of yogurt with Live and Active Cultures provide your body with an excellent source of gut-friendly probiotics. Don't fall for the false marketing on low-fat yogurts)

Digest-ability (full fat, less-processed, organic versions are more easily recognized by our bodies, and also contain the enzymes our bodies need to digest dairy in the first place)

Resources/References

Chapter 1:

Séralini, G.-E., Clair, E., Mesnage, R., Gress, S., Defarge, N., Malatesta, M., ... de Vendômois, J. S. (2014). Republished study: long-term toxicity of a Roundup herbicide and a Roundup-tolerant genetically modified maize. Environmental Sciences Europe, 26(1), 14. http://doi.org/10.1186/s12302-014-0014-5

Autism Spectrum Disorder. (2017). Centers for Disease Control & Prevention. "Data & Statistics." https://www.cdc.gov/ncbddd/autism/data.html

Weir HK, Anderson RN, Coleman King SM, Soman A, Thompson TD, Hong Y, et al. Heart Disease and Cancer Deaths — Trends and Projections in the United States, 1969–2020. Prev Chronic Dis 2016;13:160211. DOI: http://dx.doi.org/10.5888/pcd13.160211.

The National Institute of Diabetes and Digestive and Kidney Diseases Health Information Center. (2017). Overweight & Obesity Statistics. https://www.niddk.nih.gov/health-information/health-statistics/overweight-obesity

Centers for Disease Control & Prevention. 2017. Diabetes. Fact Sheets. https://www.cdc.gov/diabetes/library/factsheets.html

Diabetes Care report: "The Economic Burden of Elevated Blood Glucose Levels in 2012: Diagnosed and Undiagnosed Diabetes, Gestational Diabetes Mellitus, and Prediabetes" (December 2014)

Laborde Debucquet, David; Bizikova, Livia; Lallemant, Tess; Smaller, Carin. 2016. Ending hunger: What would it cost? Winnipeg, Manitoba, Canada: International Institute for Sustainable Development (IISD). http://www.iisd.org/sites/default/files/publications/ending-hunger-what-would-it-cost.pdf

Any Mental Illness (AMI) Among Adults. (n.d.). Retrieved October 23, 2015, from http://www.nimh.nih.gov/health/statistics/prevalence/any-mental-illness-ami-among-adults.shtml

Pratt, L. Brody, D., Gu, Q. 2011. Antidepressant Use in Persons Aged 12 and Over: United States, 2005–2008. Centers for Disease Control & Prevention. https://www.cdc.gov/nchs/products/databriefs/db76.htm.

Alzheimer's Association. 2017. Alzheimer's Disease Facts & Figures. https://www.alz.org/facts/

Collier, C., Harper, J., Cantrell, W., Wang, W., Foster, K., Elewski, B. 2008. The prevalence of acne in adults 20 years and older. Journal of the American Academy of Dermatology. https://doi.org/10.1016/j.jaad.2007.06.045

Lucintel. 2016. Growth Opportunities in the Global Skincare Product Industry. https://www.marketresearch.com/Lucintel-v2747/Growth-Opportunities-Global-Skincare-Product-10497687/?progid=89498

Asthma & Allergy Foundation of America. 2017. Allergy Facts & Figures. http://www.aafa.org/page/allergy-facts.aspx

American Academy of Allergy Asthma & Immunology. 2017. Allergy Statistics. http://www.aaaai.org/about-aaaai/newsroom/allergy-statistics

Chapter 2:

Séralini, G.-E., Clair, E., Mesnage, R., Gress, S., Defarge, N., Malatesta, M., … de Vendômois, J. S. (2014). Republished study: long-term toxicity of a Roundup herbicide and a Roundup-tolerant genetically modified maize. Environmental Sciences Europe, 26(1), 14. http://doi.org/10.1186/s12302-014-0014-5

Chapter 3:

Smits SA1, Leach J2,3, Sonnenburg ED1, Gonzalez CG4, Lichtman JS4, Reid G5, Knight R6, Manjurano A7, Changalucha J7, Elias JE4, Dominguez-Bello MG8, Sonnenburg JL1. (2017). Seasonal cycling in the gut microbiome of the Hadza hunter-gatherers of Tanzania. Science. ;357(6353):802-806. doi: 10.1126/science.aan4834.

Chapter 4:

Bischoff, S. C., Barbara, G., Buurman, W., Ockhuizen, T., Schulzke, J.-D., Serino, M., … Wells, J. M. (2014). Intestinal permeability – a new target for disease prevention and therapy. BMC Gastroenterology, 14, 189. http://doi.org/10.1186/s12876-014-0189-7

Fasano A, Berti I, Gerarduzzi T, Not T, Colletti RB, Drago S, Elitsur Y, Green PHR, Guandalini S, Hill ID, Pietzak M, Ventura A, Thorpe M, Kryszak D, Fornaroli F, Wasserman SS, Murray JA, Horvath K. (2003). Prevalence of Celiac Disease in At-Risk and Not-At-Risk Groups in the United States Large Multicenter Study. Arch Intern Med. 163(3):286–292. doi:10.1001/archinte.163.3.286

Rodrigo, Luis & Fuentes, D & Riestra, Sabino & Niño, P & Alvarez, Noemí & Lopez Vazquez, Antonio & López-Larrea, C. (2007). Increased prevalence of celiac disease in first-grade relatives: A report of a family with 19 studied members. Revista española de enfermedades digestivas : organo oficial de la Sociedad Española de Patología Digestiva. 99. 149-55.

Chapter 5:

Bischoff, S. C., Barbara, G., Buurman, W., Ockhuizen, T., Schulzke, J.-D., Serino, M., ... Wells, J. M. (2014). Intestinal permeability – a new target for disease prevention and therapy. BMC Gastroenterology, 14, 189. http://doi.org/10.1186/s12876-014-0189-7

Hsiang-Yao Shih, Deng-Chyang Wu, Wan-Ting Huang, Yong-Yu Chang, Fang-Jung Yu, Glutaraldehyde-induced colitis: Case reports and literature review, The Kaohsiung Journal of Medical Sciences, Volume 27, Issue 12, 2011, Pages 577-580, ISSN 1607-551X, http://dx.doi.org/10.1016/j.kjms.2011.06.036.

Tursi A, Elisei W, Picchio M, Brandimarte G. (2014). Increased faecal calprotectin predicts recurrence of colonic diverticulitis. International Journal of Colorectal Disease. 29(8):931-5. doi: 10.1007/s00384-014-1884-0.

The American Institute of Stress. 2017. https://www.stress.org/americas-1-health-problem/ (Citing: America's Leading Adult Health Problem, by Paul J. Rosch, M.D., F.A.C.P., in USA Magazine, May 1991; American Academy of Family Physicians Survey, 1988; U.S. News & World Report, December 11, 1995; Perkins (1994), Harvard Business Review)

Chapter 6:

Johns Hopkins Medicine. (2018, February 1). Bacteria play critical role in driving colon cancers. ScienceDaily.www.sciencedaily.com/releases/2018/02/180201173406.htm

Gopalakrishnan, V. et al. (2017). Potential role of intratumor bacteria in mediating tumor resistance to the chemotherapeutic drug gemcitabine. Science. 357 (6356): 1156-1160. http://dx.doi.org/10.1126/science.aan4236

Hullar MA1, Burnett-Hartman AN, Lampe JW. (2014). Gut microbes, diet, and cancer. Cancer Treatment Research. 159:377-99. doi: 10.1007/978-3-642-38007-5_22..

Hoban, A., Stilling, R., Moloney, G., Moloney, R., Shanahan, F., Dinan, T., Cryan, J., Clarke, G. (2017). Microbial regulation of microRNA expression in the amygdala and prefrontal cortex. Microbiome 5:102. https://microbiomejournal.biomedcentral.com/articles/10.1186/s40168-017-0321-3

Aarts, E., Ederveen, T., Naaijen, J., Zwiers, M., Boerkhorst, J., Timmerman, H., Smeekens, S., Netea, M., Buitelaar, J., Franke, B., van Hijim, S., Vasquez, A. (2017). Gut microbiome in ADHD and its relation to neural reward anticipation. PLOS One. https://doi.org/10.1371/journal.pone.0183509

Borgo, F., Riva, A., Benetti, A., Casiraghi, MC, Bertelli, S., Garbossa, S., Anselmetti, S., Scarone, S., Pontiroli, A., Morace, G., Borghi, E. (2017). Microbiota in anorexia nervosa: The triangle between bacterial species, metabolites and psychological tests. PLOS One. https://doi.org/10.1371/journal.pone.0179739

Simonyte Sjödin, Kotryna; Vidman, Linda; Rydén, Patrik; West, Christina E. (2016). Emerging evidence of the role of gut microbiota in the development of allergic diseases. Current Opinion in Allergy and Clinical Immunology: 16 (4): 390-395. doi: 10.1097/ACI.0000000000000277

Fujimura KE, Sitarik AR, Havstad S, Lin DL, Levan S, Fadrosh D, Panzer AR, LaMere B, Rackaityte E, Lukacs NW, Wegienka G, Boushey HA, Ownby DR, Zoratti EM, Levin AM, Johnson CC, Lynch SV. (2016). Neonatal gut microbiota associates with childhood multisensitized atopy and T cell differentiation. Natural Medicine. doi: 10.1038/nm.4176.

University of Illinois College of Agricultural, Consumer and Environmental Sciences. (2017). Gut microbes may talk to the brain through cortisol. ScienceDaily. from www.sciencedaily.com/releases/2017/08/170821122736.htm

Baker, J. et al. (2017). Estrogen–gut microbiome axis: Physiological and clinical implications. Maturitas: The European Menopause Journal. DOI: https://doi.org/10.1016/j.maturitas.2017.06.025

Technical University of Denmark (DTU). (2016). Gut bacteria affect our metabolism. ScienceDaily. www.sciencedaily.com/releases/2016/11/161121094111.htm

Menni, C., Jackson, MA, Pallister, T., Steves, CJ, Spector, TD, Valdes, AM., (2017). Gut microbiome diversity and high-fibre intake are related to lower long-term weight gain. Journal of Obesity. 41, 1099-1105. doi:10.1038/ijo.2017.66

Devaraj, S., Hemarajata, P., & Versalovic, J. (2013). The Human Gut Microbiome and Body Metabolism: Implications for Obesity and Diabetes. Clinical Chemistry, 59(4), 617–628. http://doi.org/10.1373/clinchem.2012.187617

P Lu, C P Sodhi, Y Yamaguchi, H Jia, T Prindle, W B Fulton, A Vikram, K J Bibby, M J Morowitz, D J Hackam. Intestinal epithelial Toll-like receptor 4 prevents metabolic syndrome by regulating interactions between microbes and intestinal epithelial cells in mice. Mucosal Immunology, 2018; DOI: 10.1038/mi.2017.114

Mori, K. (2012). Does the gut microbiota trigger Hashimoto's thyroiditis?

Discovery Medicine; Discovery Med 14(78): 321-326. https://www.ncbi.nlm.nih.gov/pubmed/23200063

Lauritano, EC., Bilotta, AL., Emidio, MG., Lupascu, SA., Marialuisa, AL., Sottili, NS., Giovanni, MS., Gasbarrini, CG., Pontecorvi, A., Gasbarrini, A. (2007). Association between Hypothyroidism and Small Intestinal Bacterial Overgrowth.The Journal of Clinical Endocrinology & Metabolism, 92 (11): 4180–4184, https://doi.org/10.1210/jc.2007-0606

Serino, M., Blasco-Baque, V., Nicolas, S., & Burcelin, R. (2014). Far from the Eyes, Close to the Heart: Dysbiosis of Gut Microbiota and Cardiovascular Consequences. Current Cardiology Reports, 16(11), 540. http://doi.org/10.1007/s11886-014-0540-1

Fransen, F., van Beek, A., Borghuis, T., El Aidy, S., Hugenholtz, F., van der Gaast – de Jongh, C., Savelkoul, H., De Jonge, MI, Boekschoten, M., Smidt, H., Faas, M., de Vos., P. (2017). Aged Gut Microbiota Contributes to Systemical Inflammaging after Transfer to Germ-Free Mice. Frontiers in Immunology; 10 (10):1187-1191.DOI: 10.3389/fimmu.2017.01385

Keys, A., Brozek, J., Henshel, A., Mickelson, O., & Taylor, H.L. (1950). The biology of human starvation, (Vols. 1–2). Minneapolis, MN: University of Minnesota Press.

Kalm, L.M., & Semba, R.D. (2005). They starved so that others be better fed: Remembering Ancel Keys and the Minnesota Experiment. Journal of Nutrition, 135, 1347–1352.

McGrice, M., & Porter, J. (2017). The Effect of Low Carbohydrate Diets on Fertility Hormones and Outcomes in Overweight and Obese Women: A Systematic Review. Nutrients, 9(3), 204. http://doi.org/10.3390/nu9030204

Beier, A., Hahn, V., Bornscheuer, U. T., & Schauer, F. (2014). Metabolism of alkenes and ketones by Candida maltosa and related yeasts. AMB Express, 4, 75. http://doi.org/10.1186/s13568-014-0075-2

Yau, Y. H. C., & Potenza, M. N. (2013). Stress and Eating Behaviors. Minerva Endocrinologica, 38(3), 255–267. https://www.ncbi.nlm.nih.gov/pmc/articles/PMC4214609/

Psychology of Eating. 2013. The Metabolic Power of Pleasure. The Psychology of Eating Institute. http://psychologyofeating.com/metabolic-power-pleasure/

Scelzo, A., Di Somma, S., Antonini, P., Montross, L., Schork, N., Brenner, D., & Jeste, D. (2018). Mixed-methods quantitative–qualitative study of 29 nonagenarians and centenarians in rural Southern Italy: Focus on positive psychological traits. International Psychogeriatrics, 30(1), 31-38. doi:10.1017/S1041610217002721

Jang-Young,K., Dhananjay, Y, Song Vogue, A., Sang-Baek, K., Jong Taek, P., Junghan, Y., Byung-Su, Y., Seung-Hwan, L. (2015). A prospective study of total sleep duration and incident metabolic syndrome: the ARIRANG study. Sleep Medicine. 16 (12): 1511-1515. DOI: https://doi.org/10.1016/j.sleep.2015.06.024.

Nielson Total Audience Report: Quarter 1. 2016. http://www.nielsen.com/us/en/insights/reports/2016/the-total-audience-report-q1-2016.html?afflt=ntrt15340001&afflt_uid=HHqB12FnbKg.qG7FuRWxqknC27B8uPRnrH__RQWt60TY&afflt_uid_2=AFFLT_ID_2.

Phipps-Nelson, Redman JR, Dijk DJ, Rajaratnam SM. (2003). Daytime exposure to bright light, as compared to dim light, decreases sleepiness and improves psychomotor vigilance performance. Sleep. 26(6):695-700. https://www.ncbi.nlm.nih.gov/pubmed/14572122

JustStand.org. (2017). The Facts. http://www.juststand.org/the-facts/

Brown, S. 2010. Play: How it Shapes the Brain, Opens the Imagination, and Invigorates the Soul. Penguin Books, Ltd.

Brussoni, M., Olsen, L. L., Pike, I., & Sleet, D. A. (2012). Risky Play and Children's Safety: Balancing Priorities for Optimal Child Development. International Journal of Environmental Research and Public Health, 9(9), 3134–3148. http://doi.org/10.3390/ijerph9093134

Dreisbach, S. (2014). How do you feel about your body? Glamour. https://www.glamour.com/story/body-image-how-do-you-feel-about-your-body.

Andreassen, C. S., Pallesen, S., & Griffiths, M. D. (2017). The relationship between addictive use of social media, narcissism, and self-esteem: Findings from a large national survey. Addictive Behaviors, 64, 287-293. doi:10.1016/j.addbeh.2016.03.006

Deloitte. (2016). Global Mobile Consumer Survey: U.S. Edition. https://www2.deloitte.com/us/en/pages/technology-media-and-telecommunications/articles/global-mobile-consumer-survey-us-edition.html?id=us:el:pr:gmcs:awa:tmt:120915c

Saiidi, U. (2015). Social media making millennials less social: Study. CNBC. https://www.cnbc.com/2015/10/15/social-media-making-millennials-less-social-study.html

Egolf, B., Lasker, J., Wolf, S. & Potvin, L. 1992. The Roseto Effect: A 50-Year Comparison of Mortality Rates. American Journal of Public Health.

Ertel, M., Glymour, M., Berkman, L. (2009). Social networks and health: A life course perspective integrating observational and experimental evidence. Journal of Social & Personal Relationships. 26 (1): 73-92.

Everson-Rose, S. Lewis, T. (2005). Psychological Factors Affecting Cardiovascular Disease. Annual Review of

Public Health. 26:469-500. https://doi.org/10.1146/annurev.publhealth.26.021304.144542

Robles, T., Glaser, J. (2003). The physiology of marriage: pathways to health. 79 (3): 409-416. Physiology & Behavior. https://doi.org/10.1016/S0031-9384(03)00160-4.

Uchio, BN. (2006). Social support and health: a review of physiological processes potentially underlying links to disease outcomes. Journal of Behavioral Medicine. 29 (4): 377-87. https://www.ncbi.nlm.nih.gov/pubmed/16758315

Egolf, B., Lasker, J., Wolf, S., & Potvin, L. (1992). The Roseto effect: a 50-year comparison of mortality rates. American Journal of Public Health, 82(8), 1089–1092. https://www.ncbi.nlm.nih.gov/pmc/articles/PMC1695733/

Kagamimori, S., Nasermoaddeli, A., & Wang, H. (2004). Psychosocial stressors in inter-human relationships and health at each life stage: A review. Environmental Health and Preventive Medicine, 9(3), 73-86. doi:10.1265/ehpm.9.73

Benesh, M. (2016). Under New Safety Law, 20 Toxic Chemicals EPA Should Act on Now: What the New Chemical Law Will Do. Environmental Working Group. https://www.ewg.org/research/under-new-safety-law-20-toxic-chemicals-epa-should-act-now/what-new-chemical-safety-law#.WpNF-maZPwd

Kwa M, Welty LJ, Xu S. Adverse Events Reported to the US Food and Drug Administration for Cosmetics and Personal Care Products. JAMA Intern Med. Published online June 26, 2017. doi:10.1001/jamainternmed.2017.276

CDC. (2010). Exposure to Environmental Toxins. https://www.cdc.gov/breastfeeding/disease/environmental_toxins.htm

Maier, Lisa & Pruteanu, Mihaela & Kuhn, Michael & Zeller, Georg & Telzerow, Anja & Erin Anderson, Exene & Rita Brochado, Ana

& Conrad Fernandez, Keith & Dose, Hitomi & Mori, Hirotada & Patil, Kiran & Bork, Peer & Typas, Athanasios. (2018). Extensive impact of non-antibiotic drugs on human gut bacteria. Nature. DOI: 10.1038/nature25979. https://www.nature.com/articles/nature25979

Yeojun Yun, Han-Na Kim, Song E Kim, Yoosoo Chang, Seungho Ryu, Hocheol Shin, So-Youn Woo, Hyung-Lae Kim. (2017). The Effect of Probiotics, Antibiotics, and Antipyretic Analgesics on Gut Microbiota Modification. JOURNAL OF BACTERIOLOGY AND VIROLOGY, 47(1), 64-74.

Shou K., Yan Hui, Jiang Tao, Guo Chun Y., Liu Jing J., Dong Shuang Z., Yang Kai L., Wang Ya J., Cao Zhi J., Li Sheng L. (2017). Preparing the Gut with Antibiotics Enhances Gut Microbiota Reprogramming Efficiency by Promoting Xenomicrobiota Colonization. Frontiers in Microbiology. 8: 1208. DOI=10.3389/fmicb.2017.01208.

Bercik P1, Denou E, Collins J, Jackson W, Lu J, Jury J, Deng Y, Blennerhassett P, Macri J, McCoy KD, Verdu EF, Collins SM. 2011. The intestinal microbiota affect central levels of brain-derived neurotropic factor and behavior in mice. Gastroenterology. https://www.ncbi.nlm.nih.gov/pubmed/21683077

Juth, V., Smyth, J. M., & Santuzzi, A. M. (2008). How Do You Feel? Self-esteem Predicts Affect, Stress, Social Interaction, and Symptom Severity during Daily Life in Patients with Chronic Illness. Journal of Health Psychology, 13(7), 884–894. http://doi.org/10.1177/1359105308095062

Konturek PC, Brzozowski T, Konturek SJ. 2011. Stress and the gut: pathophysiology, clinical consequences, diagnostic approach and treatment options. Journal of Physiology and Pharmacology. http://www.jpp.krakow.pl/journal/archive/12_11/pdf/591_12_11_article.pdf

Hosseinzadeh, S. T., Poorsaadati, S., Radkani, B., & Forootan, M. (2011). Psychological disorders in patients with chronic constipation. Gastroenterology and Hepatology From Bed to Bench, 4(3), 159–163.

Jessurun, J. G., van Harten, P. N., Egberts, T. C. G., Pijl, Y. J., Wilting, I., & Tenback, D. E. (2016). The Relation between Psychiatric Diagnoses and Constipation in Hospitalized Patients: A Cross-Sectional Study. Psychiatry Journal, 2016, 2459693. http://doi.org/10.1155/2016/2459693

Vlieger, A. M., Rutten, Juliette M T M, Govers, Anita M A P, Frankenhuis, C., & Benninga, M. A. (2012). Long-term follow-up of gut-directed hypnotherapy vs. standard care in children with functional abdominal pain or irritable bowel syndrome. The American Journal of Gastroenterology, 107(4), 627. doi:10.1038/ajg.2011.487

Dwivedi, S. K., & Kotnala, A. (2014). Impact of hypnotherapy in mitigating the symptoms of depression. Indian Journal Of Positive Psychology, 5(4), 456-460.

Ballou, S., & Keefer, L. (2017). Psychological interventions for irritable bowel syndrome and inflammatory bowel diseases. Clinical and Translational Gastroenterology, 8(1), e214. doi:10.1038/ctg.2016.69

Emmanuel, A., Mason, H., & Kamm, M. (2001). Relationship between psychological state and level of activity of extrinsic gut innervation in patients with a functional gut disorder. Gut, 49(2), 209–213. http://doi.org/10.1136/gut.49.2.209

Clifton, J. (2017). The World's Broken Workplace. Gallup. http://news.gallup.com/opinion/chairman/212045/world-broken-workplace.aspx?g_source=position1&g_medium=related&g_campaign=tiles

Bureau of Labor Statistics. (2017). Average hours employed people spent working on days worked by day of week. American Time Use Survey. https://www.bls.gov/charts/american-time-use/emp-by-ftpt-job-edu-h.htm

Pressman, S. D., Matthews, K. A., Cohen, S., Martire, L. M., Scheier, M., Baum, A., & Schulz, R. (2009). Association of Enjoyable Leisure Activities With Psychological and Physical Well-Being. Psychosomatic Medicine, 71(7), 725–732. http://doi.org/10.1097/PSY.0b013e3181ad7978

Lufityanto, G., Donkin, C., & Pearson, J. (2016). Measuring Intuition: Nonconscious Emotional Information Boosts Decision Accuracy and Confidence. Psychological Science. doi: 10.1177/0956797616629403

Kelly, A.,Wang, L. & Gondoli, D. (2012) Life without Lies: Can Living More. Honestly Improve Health? Anita E. Kelly. Lijuan Wang. Department of Psychology. University of Notre Dame. Page 2. " Science of Honesty" project 2011-2013. https://cbsphilly.files.wordpress.com/2012/08/kelly-a-life-without-lies.pdf

Enck, P., Horing, B., Weimer, K., & Klosterhalfen, S. (2012). Placebo responses and placebo effects in functional bowel disorders. European Journal of Gastroenterology & Hepatology, 24(1), 1-8. 10.1097/MEG.0b013e32834bb951

Whorwell PJ; Prior A; Faragher EB. Controlled trial of hypnotherapy in the treatment of severe refractory irritable-bowel syndrome.The Lancet 1984, 2: 1232-4. DOI: https://doi.org/10.1016/S0140-6736(84)92793-4

Pitz M, Cheang M, Bernstein CN. 2005. Defining the predictors of the placebo response in irritable bowel syndrome. Clin. Gastroenterol. Hepatol; 3: 237–47.

Sirois, F. M., Kitner, R., & Hirsch, J. K. (2015). Self-compassion, affect, and health-promoting behaviors. Health Psychology, 34(6), 661-669.

http://dx.doi.org/10.1037/hea0000158

Chapter 7B:

Hirshkowitz, M, et al. 2015. National Sleep Foundation's sleep time duration recommendations: methodology and results summary. Sleep Health. 1(1):40-43. doi: 10.1016/j.sleh.2014.12.010.

Williamson AM, Feyer A. 2000. Moderate sleep deprivation produces impairments in cognitive and motor performance equivalent to legally prescribed levels of alcohol intoxication Occupational and Environmental Medicine. 57:649-655.

Chapter 7C:

Brown SR, Cann PA, Read NW. 1990. Effect of coffee on distal colon function.Gut. 31:450-453. http://dx.doi.org/10.1136/gut.31.4.450.

Cheat Sheet Protocols

SIBO

Chedid, V., Dhalla, S., Clarke, J. O., Roland, B. C., Dunbar, K. B., Koh, J., ... Mullin, G. E. (2014). Herbal Therapy Is Equivalent to Rifaximin for the Treatment of Small Intestinal Bacterial Overgrowth. Global Advances in Health and Medicine, 3(3), 16–24. http://doi.org/10.7453/gahmj.2014.019

Brown, K., Scott-Hoy, B., & Jennings, L. W. (2016). Response of irritable bowel syndrome with constipation patients administered a combined quebracho/conker tree/M. balsamea Willd extract. World Journal of Gastrointestinal Pharmacology and Therapeutics, 7(3), 463–468. http://doi.org/10.4292/wjgpt.v7.i3.463

a combined quebracho/conker tree/M. balsamea Willd extract. World Journal of Gastrointestinal Pharmacology and Therapeutics, 7(3), 463–468. http://doi.org/10.4292/wjgpt.v7.i3.463

Author Bio:
Dr. Lauryn Lax, OTD, NTP

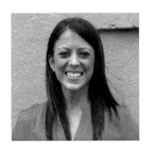

Dr. Lauryn Lax is a Doctor of Occupational Therapy, Nutritional Therapy Practitioner, Functional Medicine Practitioner, author and speaker, with over 20 years of clinical and personal experience specializing in gut health, intuitive eating, disordered eating, anxiety, hormone balance and women's health. She is a published journalist and speaker, and her work has been featured in Oxygen Magazine, Women's Health, Paleo Magazine, Breaking Muscle, CrossFit Inc, USA Today, ABC and CBS News. She lives in Austin and operates a virtual Functional Medicine practice, Thrive Wellness & Recovery, LLC, working with clients and patients around the world to get unstuck from their health, food, mindset and fitness ruts.

Who Am I?
- Doctor of Occupational Therapy (Belmont University)
- Nutritional Therapy Practitioner (Nutritional Therapy Association)
- Functional Medicine Practitioner (Institute for Functional Medicine (AFMCP), Kresser Institute)
- B.A. Journalism/Communications (University of Texas)
- Certified Fitness Professional (ACE, CrossFit Level I)

What Do I Do?
- Functional Medicine
- Nutritional Therapy
- Counseling, Coaching & Occupational Therapy
- Eating Disorder Recovery Coaching

The Real Me:
- I love mornings
- Mondays are my favorite day of the week
- Julia Roberts (actress) and I share the same birthday
- As a kid, I wanted to be a writer and the "next" Katie Couric on the Today Show
- My biggest pet peeves are wasting time and traffic
- Country and boy-band music from the 90's gets me singing and dancing
- I grew up in Arkansas
- Austin, Texas is my favorite place on earth
- I pick the beach over mountains any day!
- I love volunteering with kids and visiting older people in the nursing home
- I have an Amazon Prime addiction (I love reading new books!)

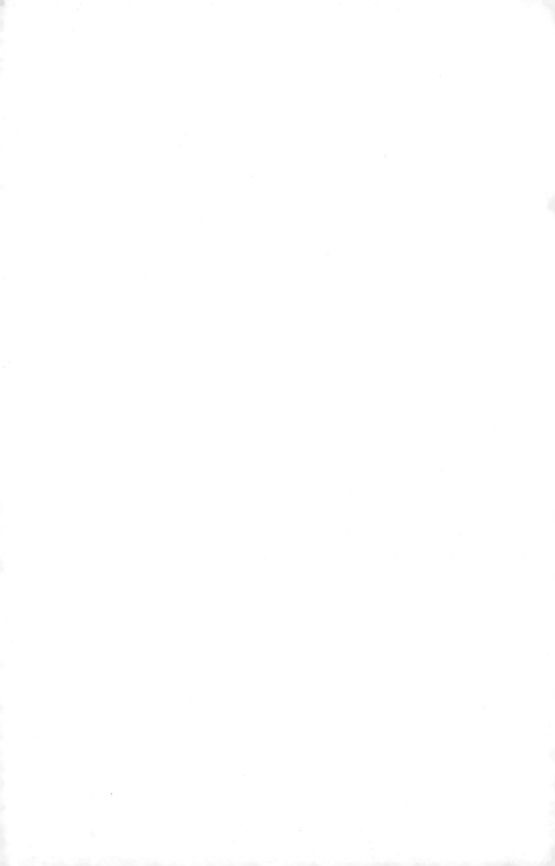

Made in United States
North Haven, CT
15 May 2022